Cardiovascular

DATE DUE

8/31/23 ILL			

D1296094

To R and K

—My constant companions

AV

To Indigo Lucy

—May the wonder of nature always fascinate you

DJP

For Elsevier
Commissioning Editor: Laurence Hunter
Development Editor: Helen Leng
Project Manager: Elouise Ball
Design Direction: Erik Bigland
Illustration Manager: Merlyn Harvey
Illustrator: Paul Bernson

Cardiovascular Magnetic Resonance Made Easy

Edited by:

Anitha Varghese BSc MRCP

Research Fellow, Royal Brompton Hospital, London; Specialist Register in Cardiology, West Midlands Deanery, UK

Dudley J Pennell MD FRCP FACC FESC

Professor of Cardiology, National Heart and Lung Institute, Imperial College, London; Director, CMR Unit, Royal Brompton Hospital, London, UK

CHURCHILL
LIVINGSTONE

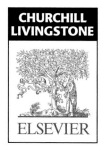

ELSEVIER

EDINBURGH LONDON NEW YORK OXFORD PHILADELPHIA ST LOUIS SYDNEY TORONTO 2008

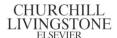

CHURCHILL LIVINGSTONE
ELSEVIER

An imprint of Elsevier Limited

© 2008, Elsevier Limited. All rights reserved.

The right of Anitha Varghese and Dudley J Pennell to be identified as editors of this work has been asserted by them in accordance with the Copyright, Designs and Patents Act 1988.

First published 2008

ISBN-13: 978-0-443103-018

British Library Cataloguing in Publication Data
A catalogue record for this book is available from the British Library

Library of Congress Cataloging in Publication Data
A catalog record for this book is available from the Library of Congress

Notice

Knowledge and best practice in this field are constantly changing. As new research and experince broaden our knowledge, changes in practice, treatment and drug therapy may become necessary or appropriate. Readers are advised to check the most current information provided (i) on procedures featured or (ii) by the manufacturer of each product to be administered, to verify the recommended dose or formula, the method and duration of administration, and contraindications. It is the responsibility of the practitioner, relying on their own experience and knowledge of the patient, to make diagnoses, to determine dosages and the best treatment for each individual patient, and to take all appropriate safety precautions. To the fullest extent of the law, neither the publisher nor the authors assume any liability for any injury and/or damage to persons or property arising out of or related to any use of the material contained in this book.

The Publisher

Working together to grow libraries in developing countries

www.elsevier.com | www.bookaid.org | www.sabre.org

ELSEVIER   BOOK AID International   Sabre Foundation

---

your source for books, journals and multimedia in the health sciences

www.elsevierhealth.com

The publisher's policy is to use **paper manufactured from sustainable forests**

Preface

Cardiovascular magnetic resonance (CMR) describes the use of magnetic resonance imaging (MRI) for the anatomical and functional evaluation of the heart and vascular tree. The traditional arsenal of noninvasive imaging modalities available to the cardiologist and cardiothoracic surgeon include echocardiography and nuclear cardiology. CMR is a contemporary and complementary technology which is rapidly gaining popularity in this dynamic field.

At present, there are several large reference books on CMR which provide a comprehensive guide to the physics and clinical application of this technique. In this book we provide a more easily digestible synopsis which is readily portable and can be rapidly updated. The Royal Brompton Hospital has been at the vanguard of CMR throughout its journey from a fledgling research idea to fully grown clinical ideal and we hope this small book successfully condenses our experience in this arena.

We have targeted the text predominantly at the needs of cardiologists and cardiothoracic surgeons wishing to acquaint themselves with CMR — what it can do and what it cannot. The chapters therefore concentrate on the cardiac side of CMR but also address its more established vascular uses in a later section. Before both of these, however, we outline some of the basic principles of MRI.

Anitha Varghese
Dudley Pennell

Acknowledgements

Our thanks go to all the past and present members of the CMR Department, Royal Brompton Hospital. Additionally, we express our specific gratitude to Laurence Hunter, Helen Leng, Charles Lauder Jr and Elouise Ball at Elsevier, Ritesh Mewar, Didier Locca, Henning Steen, Taigang He, Paul Kotwinski and Karen Symmonds for their role in the preparation of the final manuscript.

Note to readers

Please note that the statements made in this book refer to CMR performed at a magnet field strength of 1.5 Tesla.

Contributors

Beatriz Bouzas MD
Consultant Cardiologist, Servicio de
Cardiologia, Complejo Hospitalario
Universitario Juan Canalejo, La Caruña, Spain

Ping Chai MRCP
Consultant Cardiologist, Cardiac
Department, National University Hospital,
Singapore
The Heart Institute, National Healthcare
Group, Singapore

Ilse Crevits MD
General Radiologist, HHR—Site Roeselare
Hospital, Roeselare
Visiting Consultant CMR, University
Hospitals of Leuven, Belgium

George E Gentchos MD
Assistant Professor of Radiology, College of
Medicine University of Vermont, Burlington,
Vermont, USA

Chad A Hoyt MD FACC
Director of Cardiovascular CT and MR,
Stroobants Heart Center, Centra Health
Director of Noninvasive Cardiovascular
Services, Bedford Memorial Hospital
Cardiologist, The Cardiovascular Group,
Centra Health, Lynchburg, Virginia, USA

Katharina Kiss MD
Department of Cardiology, Hospital
of Hietzing, City of Vienna and
Cardiovascular Imaging Unit
Rudolfinerhaus Vienna, Austria

James C Moon MA MRCP MD
Senior Lecturer in Cardiology, The Heart
Hospital, London, UK

Richard Steeds MA MRCP MD
Consultant Cardiologist with Special
Interest in Imaging, University Hospital
Birmingham NHS Foundation Trust,
Birmingham, UK

Marc D Tischler BA MD FACC FAHA FACP
Associate Professor of Medicine, University
of Vermont College of Medicine
Director, Cardiac Ultrasound Laboratory,
Fletcher Allen Health Care
Director, Clinical Cardiac MR Unit, Fletcher
Allen Health Care, Canada

Anitha Varghese BSc MRCP
Research Fellow, Royal Brompton Hospital,
London; Specialist Register in Cardiology,
West Midlands Deanery, UK

Abbreviations

ACHD	Adult congenital heart disease	IVS	Interventricular septum
AFD	Anderson Fabry disease	kg	Kilograms
AICD	Automated implantable cardiac defibrillator	l/min	Litres per minute
		LA	Left atrium
AMVL	Anterior mitral valve leaflet	LAD	Left anterior descending artery
Ao	Aorta	LCx	Left circumflex artery
APVD	Anomalous pulmonary venous drainage	LGE	Late gadolinium enhancement
		LMS	Left main stem
AR	Aortic regurgitation	LPA	Left pulmonary artery
ARVC	Arrhythmogenic right ventricular cardiomyopathy	LV	Left ventricle
		LVEDV	Left ventricular end-diastolic volume
AS	Aortic stenosis		
ASD	Atrial septal defect	LVEF	Left ventricular ejection fraction
AV	Aortic valve	LVESV	Left ventricular end-systolic volume
CABG	Coronary artery bypass grafting		
CAD	Coronary artery disease	LVH	Left ventricular hypertrophy
ccTGA	Congenitally corrected transposition of the great arteries	LVNC	Left ventricular non-compaction
		LVOT	Left ventricular outflow tract
CE-MRA	Contrast-enhanced magnetic resonance angiography	LVSV	Left ventricular stroke volume
		m/s	Metres per second
CFR	Coronary flow reserve	MAPCAs	Major aortopulmonary collateral arteries
cm	Centimetres		
CMR	Cardiovascular magnetic resonance	MHz	Megahertz
		MI	Myocardial infarction
CSF	Cerebrospinal fluid	min	Minute
CT	Computed tomography	MIP	Maximal intensity projection
DCM	Dilated cardiomyopathy	mL	Millilitre(s)
DSE	Dobutamine stress echocardiography	ml/s	Millilitre per second
		mm	Millimetres
ECG	Electrocardiogram	mmHg	Millimetres of mercury
EDV	End-diastolic volume	MPA	Main pulmonary artery
EF	Ejection fraction	MPR	Multiplanar reconstruction
EGE	Early gadolinium enhancement	MR	Mitral regurgitation
ESV	End-systolic volume	MRA	Magnetic resonance angiography
FLASH	Fast low-angle shot		
FSE	Fast spin echo	MRI	Magnetic resonance imaging
g/m^2	Grams per metre squared	MRS	Magnetic resonance spectroscopy
Gd	Gadolinium		
Gd-DTPA	Gadolinium diethylenetriamine pentaacetic acid	ms	Milliseconds
		MS	Mitral stenosis
GE	Gradient echo	MV	Mitral valve
HCM	Hypertrophic cardiomyopathy	MVO	Microvascular obstruction
IAS	Interatrial septum	MVP	Mitral valve prolapse
IVC	Inferior vena cava	PA	Pulmonary artery

Abbreviations (continued)

PAPVD	Partial anomalous pulmonary venous drainage		T	Tesla
PCI	Percutaneous coronary intervention		T1W	T1-weighted/weighting
			T2W	T2-weighted/weighting
PDA	Patent ductus arteriosus		TGA	Transposition of the great arteries
PMVL	Posterior mitral valve leaflet			
PR	Pulmonary regurgitation		TOE	Transoesophageal echocardiography/ echocardiogram
PS	Pulmonary stenosis			
PV	Pulmonary valve			
RA	Right atrium		TOF	Tetralogy of Fallot
RCA	Right coronary artery		TR	Tricuspid regurgitation
RF	Radiofrequency		TS	Tricuspid stenosis
RPA	Right pulmonary artery		TSE	Turbo spin echo
RV	Right ventricle		TTE	Transthoracic echocardiography/ echocardiogram
RVH	Right ventricular hypertrophy			
RVOT	Right ventricular outflow tract			
RVSV	Right ventricular stroke volume		TV	Tricuspid valve
SE	Spin echo		Venc	Maximal encoding velocity
SNR	Signal-to-noise ratio		V_{max}	Peak velocity
SoV	Sinus of Valsalva		VSD	Ventricular septal defect
SSD	Shaded surface display		WMA	Wall motion abnormality/ abnormalities
SSFP	Steady state free precession			
SV	Stroke volume		2D	Two-dimensional
SVC	Superior vena cava		3D	Three-dimensional
			μg	Micrograms

Contents

Chapter 1

Principles of CMR

Anitha Varghese

■ Basic physics

MRI is based on *nuclear magnetic resonance*, the phenomenon of the resonance of atomic nuclei in response to radiofrequency (RF) waves. The hydrogen atom is the simplest and most abundant element in the body and consists of one proton nucleus orbited by one electron. The hydrogen nucleus can therefore also be termed a proton, and current clinical MRI techniques are based on receiving and processing RF signals from protons. Protons have a magnetic axis which is normally randomly orientated. When a magnetic field is applied, the protons align in synchrony and spin around an axis in line with the main magnetic field—this spinning is termed *precession*. The rate at which protons precess is measured by the precession frequency, which changes linearly with increasing magnetic field strengths. When protons precess in synchrony they are said to be *in-phase*. There is loss of synchrony with time, and this is also termed *out-of-phase*.

At equilibrium within a magnetic field, overall proton alignment is in the direction of the main magnetic field and they have net longitudinal magnetization. This equilibrium can be disturbed by transmission of RF energy at the precession frequency of the proton which is 63 megaHertz (MHz) for water protons at 1.5 Tesla (T)—the strength of most commercially used magnets (Figure 1.1).

The degree of proton excitation is proportional to the amplitude and duration of the RF pulse. After excitation, proton relaxation occurs as the energy is dissipated and this process is defined by two parameters known as T1 and T2. T1 relaxation times measure the time after excitation to recover the longitudinal magnetization found in the equilibrium state. Transverse magnetization decays at a rate measured by T2, which is faster than the rate of T1 recovery. T1 and T2 relaxation vary according to the environment of the hydrogen atom within tissues and imaging sequences can be designed with different preference (or weighting) to one of these relaxation parameters for tissue characterization, known as T1-weighted (T1W) and T2-weighted (T2W) acquisitions. The values for T2 are always below that of T1, and T1 represents the upper limit of T2. T1 and T2 values tend to parallel each other when proton motion is relatively random, for example in adipose tissue, which has a short T1 and T2, and free water, which has a long T1 and T2. Tissues with a more organized structure contain abundant bound water. In this case proton motion is not random, there is increased transverse decay from the exchange of energy between protons, and T2 values become shorter than those of T1.

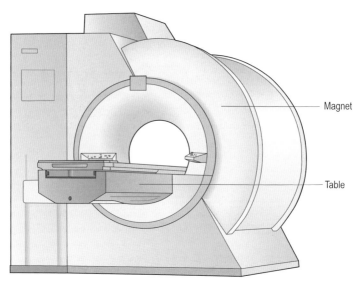

Figure 1.1 *1.5T CMR Scanner. The adjustable patient table is shown within the surrounding superconducting magnet.*

Localization of anatomical position within a selected imaging slice or volume is done with the application of frequency- and phase-encoding gradients. The corresponding direction of application of these gradients is known as the *frequency encode or phase encode direction*. With modifications of the phase-encoding gradients flowing blood can be differentiated from stationary anatomy via alterations in the phase of the MR signal. The velocity of material is proportional to the phase change or phase shift caused by its movement during gradient application.

Transmission and reception of RF energy is via special aerials known as coils with subsequent conversion of these raw data into images using ultrafast computers and a process known as Fourier transformation.

■ Main sequences

There are two fundamental types of sequence commonly used in CMR: *gradient echo* (GE) and *spin echo* (SE). As a general rule, with GE sequences both blood and fat appear white and so this technique is also known as white-blood imaging (Figure 1.2a). By contrast, in SE sequences blood is usually black but fat is white, giving rise to the term black-blood imaging (Figure 1.2b). SE sequences are more useful for anatomical imaging as opposed to the functional imaging performed with GE sequences. Variations of GE sequences are fast low-angle shot (FLASH), fast imaging with steady-state free precession (SSFP), and velocity mapping. GE imaging also forms the basis of the inversion recovery technique.

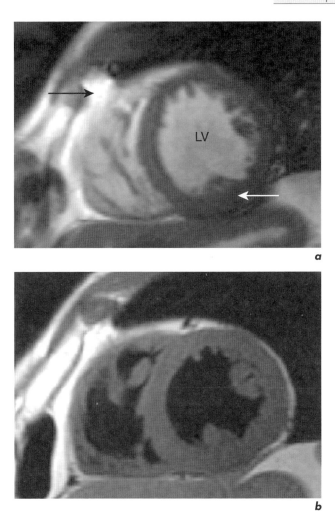

Figure 1.2 **(a)** *CMR of mid-ventricular short-axis view using GE imaging. Blood within the left ventricle (LV) is white as is the surrounding epicardial fat (black arrow). The LV myocardium (white arrow) appears mid-grey.* **(b)** *CMR in the same plane using SE imaging. Blood within the LV now appears black while the fat remains white.*

Areas of focal myocardial dysfunction and abnormal flow patterns are readily visualized with the technique of *cine imaging using SSFP* (or *cines*). Cines are obtained by rapid repetition of a variant of the basic GE sequence to obtain a series of cardiac images at progressively advancing points of the cardiac cycle which when put together form a cine loop. The weighting of SSFP sequences depends on the ratio of T2/T1, therefore most fluids and fat have a high signal and appear white. However, muscle and many other solid tissues have a long value for T1 and a short value for T2. This means that their signal intensity is reduced to shades of grey

(Figure 1.2a). In addition to cines, the SSFP sequence can also be applied as a two-dimensional (2D) single-shot technique, as a real-time technique (not requiring breath holding or electrocardiogram (ECG) triggering), and as a three-dimensional (3D) volume scan.

Velocity mapping (or *flow velocity mapping*) techniques can determine the average velocity within a single imaging voxel, typically $1 \times 1 \times 10 \, mm^3$. The operator selects the required plane and sets a maximal encoding velocity (Venc; Figure 1.3). The initial Venc used is an approximation of the velocity expected based on factors such

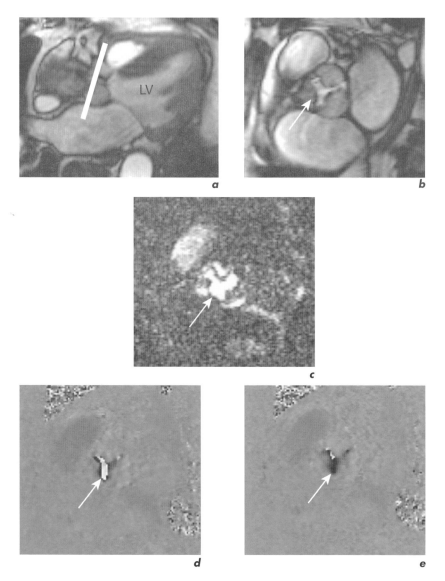

as clinical history, the type of valve or conduit lesion, and images already acquired. The Venc represents the practical upper limit of velocities that can be depicted unambiguously and should ideally be set to a numerical value just greater than the true velocity. Problems occur if it is set much higher or lower than this value—with the former leading to less sensitivity and the latter causing misrepresentation via the phenomenon of aliasing. Velocity aliasing is when the flow appears to be in the opposite direction and is characterized by a sudden transition of white-to-black or vice versa within the chosen flow region (Figure 1.3d). To eliminate or reduce aliasing a higher Venc must be set and the velocity mapping sequence repeated (Figure 1.3e). The maximal velocity of jets under interrogation should only be determined from the Venc-optimized images. Aliasing is also noted with 2D Doppler echocardiography and the technique of velocity mapping gives similar information. Subjects are asked to suspend their breathing for measurement of peak velocities using this method, which takes approximately 20 seconds to perform. An example of its use is for the quantification of peak velocity in valvular stenosis. Velocity mapping sequences are also used to calculate overall flow in a major vessel through the cardiac cycle and so can be used for quantification of regurgitation in valvular incompetence. For calculation of peak velocity and transvalvular flow, the plane used must be *through plane*—a plane perpendicular and just distal to the area of interest. Velocity mapping CMR is also used to confirm abnormal chamber communication and the ratio of pulmonary to systemic flow in shunts such as septal defects.

Compared to GE sequences, SE pulse sequences are usually more robust to system imperfections, such as magnetic field inhomogeneities. In SE imaging, structures need to be stationary for the delivery of two RF pulses. The T2 value of stationary fluid is long and gives high signal. Examples are fluid-filled structures such as cysts, which therefore appear white with SE sequences. However, flowing blood moves out of the selected slice before receiving the second pulse and so gives no signal and appears black (Figure 1.2b). Slower flowing blood can give persistent signal of varying signal intensity. Important variations of SE sequences are *fast* (or *turbo*) *spin echo* (FSE or TSE). FSE allows faster imaging than standard SE by acquiring more

Figure 1.3 *Cine images (a, b) combined with velocity mapping imaging (c–e).*
(a) Left ventricular outflow tract (LVOT) cine image of severe aortic stenosis (AS). The plane chosen for velocity mapping is just distal and perpendicular to the valve orifice (white line) and results in the oblique sagittal view shown in (b). *(b)* This shows a tricuspid aortic valve (AV; white arrow) and is the plane used for subsequent velocity mapping. AV area can be measured in this view. *(c)* Magnitude image component of the velocity mapping sequence, which confirms reduced valve area in a tricuspid AV. *(d)* The velocity mapping sequence shows systolic blood flow through the AV as black, but the Venc was set too low by the operator and the centre of the jet has turned white, a phenomenon known as aliasing (white arrow). *(e)* A second velocity mapping sequence was therefore performed using an increased Venc. The black jet through the AV is now clearly seen (white arrow) and there are only occasional edge pixels which are aliased. Peak systolic velocity in the centre of the stenotic jet was 4 m/s.

lines of data for every RF pulse delivered and allows acquisition of an entire image in a single heartbeat.

The *inversion recovery technique* uses a prepulse to create high T1 tissue contrast which is important for infarct imaging. This sequence and *contrast-enhanced magnetic resonance angiography* (CE-MRA) require use of a contrast agent. MRI contrast agents are commonly based on chelates of gadolinium which are paramagnetic, one example being gadolinium diethylenetriamine pentaacetic acid (Gd-DTPA). All gadolinium chelates currently approved for clinical use are extravascular and therefore become distributed within the interstitium following initial intravenous delivery.

CMR is performed by applying these main sequences and their variants to evaluate cardiovascular physiology and anatomy, characterize tissue, and perform vascular angiography. Additionally, cardiac metabolism can be determined with magnetic resonance spectroscopy (MRS). MRS is not covered in this book and the interested reader is referred to the further reading section.

Most CMR scans are timed with respect to the ECG (*ECG-gated*) to minimize cardiac motion artefact, and subjects are asked to suspend their breathing in end expiration (*breath-hold*) to minimize respiratory motion artefact. In some cases scans can be linked to the respiratory cycle using diaphragmatic monitoring techniques (*respiratory-gated*), allowing subjects to breathe normally (*free breathing*). High signal from fat can be reduced by the application of a frequency-selective prepulse (*fat suppression*).

Patients are advised that data are being acquired during the time when the scanner is making a noise. This noise is generated by coils within the magnet. Headphones are worn by subjects during a CMR study and this serves to minimize their discomfort during noisy periods, facilitate hearing instructions from scanner operators, and allow music to be heard throughout if requested.

■ Hardware and software requirements

CMR is performed within a large superconducting magnet with its associated radio wave generation and computer systems. Medical gases, physiological monitoring telemetry, stress infusion pumps for delivery of adenosine and dobutamine, a power injector for contrast studies, and full resuscitation equipment and drugs are also required. As mentioned above, microphones, headphones and a music system are important. Ear plugs are needed for people who are required to accompany certain patient groups such as children, and those with varying degrees of claustrophobia. Less than 2% of scans are limited by claustrophobia in the adult population and other measures of alleviating anxiety are blindfolds and prism glasses. The latter provide a way for the patient to look out even when enclosed by the bore of the magnet.

Modern scanners have ultrafast applications for real-time imaging and assessment of coronary artery disease (CAD). Additional software is important for the post-processing of data. Manufacturers such as Siemens, Philips and General Electric provide their own software for analysis and other third party packages are available such as CMRtools (Cardiovascular Imaging Solutions).

■ Imaging planes and protocols

CMR can obtain images in any plane but standard planes of reference are used to enable normal ranges to be defined. Subjects are generally scanned in the supine position and the most important planes in cardiac imaging are four-chamber, two-chamber, short-axis, LVOT and right ventricular outflow tract (RVOT). Suggested steps in obtaining these standard planes are shown sequentially in Figures 1.4–1.9, and a protocol incorporating them into routine cardiac evaluation is shown in Table 1.1.

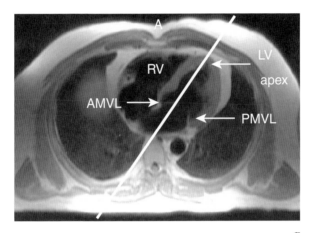

a

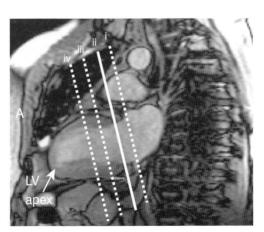

b

Figure 1.4 **(a)** *From the initial low-resolution free breathing transaxial FSE, a perpendicular* two-chamber *pilot view is obtained through a perpendicular plane placed at the mid-point of the mitral valve (MV) leaflets and the LV apex (solid white line).* **(b)** *Using this pilot two-chamber view, four perpendicular short-axial pilot views are acquired: one at the atrioventricular groove (slice ii; solid white line), and three either side on the atrial and ventricular aspects (slices i, iii and iv; dashed white lines). Abbreviations: A, anterior aspect of the image; LV, left ventricle; RV, right ventricle; AMVL, anterior mitral valve leaflet; PMVL, posterior mitral valve leaflet.*

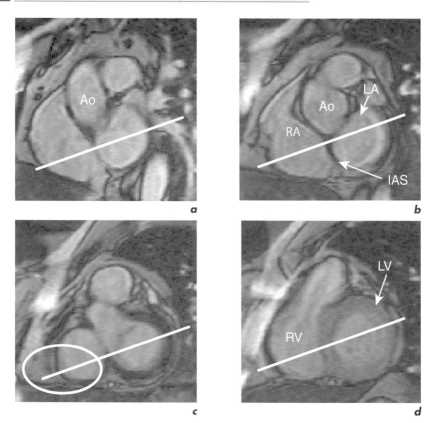

Figure 1.5 *The four-chamber cine is obtained from the resulting four short-axial pilots **(a–d)**: the imaging slab (solid white line) is placed through the centre of the LV cavity, the acute margin of the RV (c — white ellipse), and the interatrial septum (IAS), just below the aorta (Ao). LA, left atrium; RA, right atrium.*

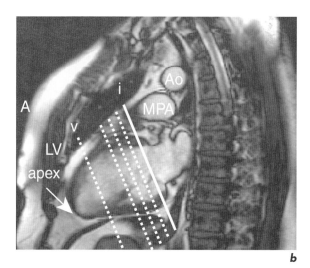

Figure 1.6 *The four-chamber cine* **(a)** *is used along with the two-chamber pilot view to obtain the two-chamber cine* **(b)***. From the end-diastolic frame of the four- and two-chamber cines, the ventricular short-axis stack of cines are acquired: the initial perpendicular short-axis slice (solid white line) is placed on the atrioventricular groove through the back of the LV and RV, and subsequent slices (dashed white lines) are acquired incrementally towards the LV apex. MPA, main pulmonary artery.*

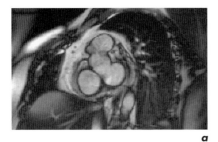

a

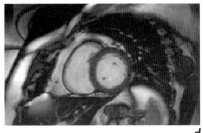

d

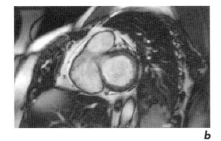

b

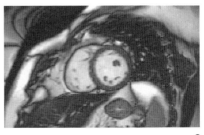

e

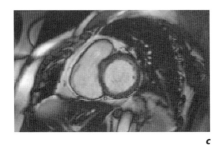

c

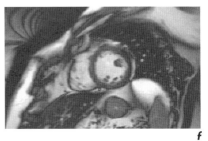

f

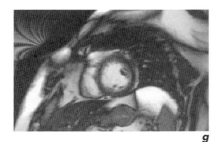

g

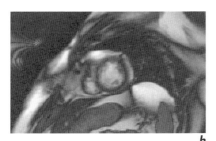

h

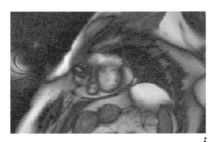

i

Figure 1.7 *Nine short-axis cines (slice thickness 7 mm, with 3 mm interslice gap) typically allows full coverage of the ventricles* **(a–i)**.

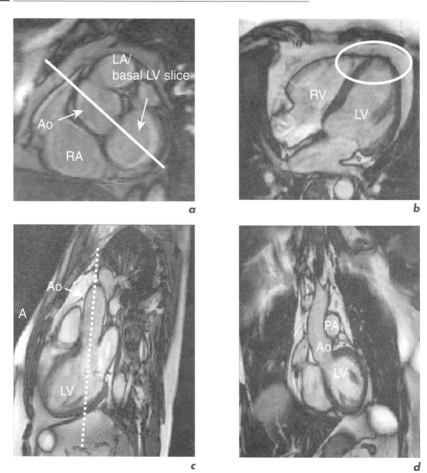

Figure 1.8 *The LVOT cine is acquired using a basal short-axis pilot* **(a)** *and four-chamber cine* **(b)***: a perpendicular slice is placed through a plane on the short-axis pilot which transects the aortic root and the distal LA/basal LV cavity (solid white line). This slice is then angulated to cut through the LV apex (white ellipse), giving the first LVOT view* **(c)***. Transection through the aorta (dashed white line) results in the second, coronal LVOT view* **(d)***. PA, pulmonary artery.*

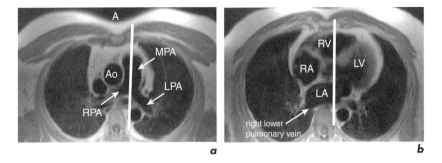

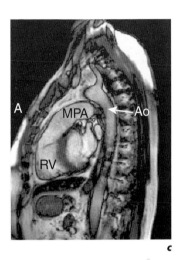

Figure 1.9 *For the RVOT cine, the transaxial FSE is recalled: a slice is placed perpendicular to the MPA, which transects the RV (**a, b**—white line). **(c)** The resulting RVOT view. RPA, right pulmonary artery; LPA, left pulmonary artery.*

Protocols for cardiac imaging involve four stages:

Stage 1: Initial, rapid, pilot scans in the three orthogonal planes—transaxial, coronal and sagittal;

Stage 2: Slower, low-resolution, comprehensive anatomical coverage from the diaphragm up to the thoracic inlet in two to three orthogonal planes—mandatory transaxial, suggested coronal, optional sagittal (mandatory in aorta imaging);

Stage 3: Specific cardiac imaging in the standard planes with GE cines and optional additional SE sequences;

Stage 4: Targeted CMR with additional planes and sequences such as inversion recovery.

Table 1.1 A standard CMR protocol which typically takes 30 minutes to perform

Pre-contrast

Five-slice SSFP pilot
Free breathing, low-resolution transaxial FSE
Breath-hold, low-resolution coronal (+ sagittal) FSE
Two-chamber pilot
Four short-axial pilots
Four-chamber and two-chamber cines
LVOT and RVOT cines
Ventricular short-axis stack cines

Post-contrast

Early gadolinium enhancement (1–5 minutes)
(a) Rpt four-chamber
(b) Rpt two-chamber
(c) Rpt LVOT
Late gadolinium enhancement (5–15 minutes)
(a) Rpt four-chamber
(b) Rpt two-chamber
(c) Rpt ventricular short-axis stack

The initial pilot images are performed in a breath-hold and are used to optimize subject placement within the magnetic field using the table-positioning tool—the centre of the heart should be at the centre of the field. The pilot scan also enables the user to check that the correct coils are activated and other system requirements are satisfactory. Subsequent low-resolution anatomical coverage using FSE acquires one image per cardiac cycle. This allows a 'quick-look' for cardiac and extracardiac pathology at the start of the study and resulting images must be reviewed prior to further acquisitions. A series of transaxial FSE images usually consists of 35–40 slices, performed in free breathing over 1–2 minutes. A 12- to 15-slice series of coronal and sagittal FSE images encompass the heart and can be performed in a breath-hold. Breath-hold images do enable more accurate positioning of subsequent slices, but respiratory variations are small within the transaxial plane. Acquisition of the standard planes has been detailed in Figures 1.4–1.9. Additional targeted planes and sequences are chosen depending on the referral request, and presence and type of other pathology.

■ Normal ranges

The normal ranges for end-diastolic volumes (EDV), end-systolic volumes (ESV), stroke volumes (SV), ejection fraction (EF) and myocardial mass indexes in males and females are presented in Table 1.2. These values are calculated using semi-automated software analysis tools applied to the ventricular short-axis stack of GE cines. Calculation of LV parameters is performed in approximately 5 minutes while

Table 1.2 Normal values for EDV, ESV, EF and myocardial mass indices in males and females

	EDV (ml)	ESV (ml)	SV (ml)	EF (%)	Mass index (g/m²)
Males					
LV	77–195	19–72	51–133	56–78	< 113
RV	88–227	23–103	52–138	47–74	< 36
Females					
LV	52–141	13–51	33–97	56–87	< 95
RV	58–154	12–68	35–98	47–80	< 33

RV parameters take longer because of the more complex anatomy. Quantification of LV parameters is mandatory for CMR reporting and RV parameters are calculated as required, for example in patients with congenital heart disease, arrhythmogenic right ventricular cardiomyopathy (ARVC), dilated cardiomyopathy (DCM) and cases of valvular regurgitation. Normal ranges are age and body surface area dependent and normatized values are also available.

Other important cardiovascular normal ranges, including dimensions for the aorta and pulmonary vessels, are currently based on echocardiographic data, since CMR specific values are yet to be published (Table 1.3).

Table 1.3 Normal ranges for cardiovascular structures by echocardiography

Cardiovascular structure	Range (cm)
Aorta dimensions (end-diastole)	
Aortic annulus	1.4–2.6
Sinus of Valsalva	2.1–3.5
Sinotubular junction	1.7–3.4
Ascending aorta (at MPA bifurcation)	2.1–3.4
Aortic arch	2.0–3.6
Descending thoracic aorta (at MPA bifurcation)	1.4–3.0
Distal descending thoracic aorta	1.3–2.8
LVOT (diastole)	1.4–2.6
RVOT (diastole)	1.8–3.4
PA dimensions (end-diastole)	
Pulmonary annulus	1.0–2.2
MPA	0.9–2.9
RPA	0.7–1.7
LPA	0.6–1.4
Venous dimensions	
Pulmonary	0.7–1.6
Inferior vena cava	1.2–2.3
Superior vena cava	0.8–2.0
Hepatic	0.5–1.1

■ Indications

The European Society of Cardiology published guidelines in November 2004 on the clinical indications for CMR (Tables 1.4–1.8) with the usefulness of this imaging technique in specific diseases classified as follows:

Class I: Provides clinically relevant information and is usually appropriate, may be used as the first-line imaging technique, usually supported by substantial literature;

Class II: Provides clinically relevant information and is frequently useful, other techniques may provide similar information, supported by limited literature;

Class III: Provides clinically relevant information but is infrequently used because information from other imaging techniques is usually adequate;

Class Inv: Potentially useful, but still investigational.

CMR also has an important role in research and development and is being increasingly used by the pharmaceutical industry in preclinical trials.

Tables 1.4, 1.5, 1.6, 1.7 and 1.8 used with kind permission of European Society of Cardiology from Pennell et al *Clinical Indications for Cardiovascular Magnetic Resonance (CMR): Consensus Panel Report*, European Heart Journal, 2004, 25 (21), 1940–1965.

Table 1.4 Indications for CMR in CAD	
Indication	**Class**
1. Assessment of global ventricular (left and right) function and mass	I
2. Detection of CAD	
Regional LV function at rest and during dobutamine stress	II
Assessment of myocardial perfusion	II
Coronary MRA (CAD)	III
Coronary MRA (anomalies)	I
Coronary MRA of bypass graft patency	II
CMR flow measurements in the coronary arteries	Inv
Arterial wall imaging	Inv
3. Acute and chronic myocardial infarction (MI)	
Detection and assessment	I
Myocardial viability	I
Ventricular septal defect	III
Mitral regurgitation (acute MI)	III
Ventricular thrombus	II
Acute coronary syndromes	Inv

Table 1.5 Indications for CMR in patients with pericardial disease, cardiac tumours, cardiomyopathies and cardiac transplants

Indication	Class
1. Pericardial effusion	III
2. Constrictive pericarditis	II
3. Detection and characterization of cardiac and pericardiac tumours	I
4. Ventricular thrombus	II
5. Hypertrophic cardiomyopathy Apical Non-apical	 I II
6. DCM Differentiation from dysfunction related to coronary artery disease	Inv I
7. ARVC	I
8. Restrictive cardiomyopathy	II
9. Siderotic cardiomyopathy (in particular thalassaemia)	I
10. Non-compaction	II
11. Post-cardiac transplantation rejection	Inv

Table 1.6 Indications for CMR in patients with valvular heart disease

Indication	Class
1. Valve morphology Bicuspic AV Other valves Vegetations	 II III Inv
2. Cardiac chamber anatomy and function	I
3. Quantification of regurgitation	I
4. Quantification of stenosis	III
5. Detection of paravalvular abscess	Inv
6. Assessment of prosthetic valves	Inv

Table 1.7 Indications for CMR in congenital heart disease

Indication	Class
General indications	
1. Initial evaluation and follow-up of adult congenital heart disease	I
Specific indications	
1. Assessment of shunt size (Qp/Qs)	I
2. Anomalies of the viscero-atrial situs	I
Isolated situs anomalies	II
Situs anomalies with complex congenital heart disease	I
3. Anomalies of the atria and venous return	
Atrial septal defect (secundum and primum)	II
Anomalous pulmonary venous return, especially in complex anomalies and cor triatriatum	I
Anomalous systemic venous return	I
Systemic or pulmonary venous obstruction following intra-atrial baffle repair or correction of anomalous pulmonary venous return	I
4. Anomalies of the atrioventricular valves	
Anatomic anomalies of the mitral and tricuspid valves	II
Functional valvular anomalies	II
Ebstein's anomaly	II
Atrioventricular septal defect	II
5. Anomalies of the ventricles	
Isolated ventricular septal defect (VSD)	III
VSD associated with complex anomalies	I
Ventricular aneurysms and diverticula	II
Supracristal VSD	I
Evaluation of right and left ventricular volumes, mass and function	I
6. Anomalies of the semilunar valves	
Isolated valvular pulmonary stenosis and valvular dysplasia	III
Supravalvular pulmonary stenosis	II
Pulmonary regurgitation	I
Isolated valvular AS	III
Subaortic stenosis	III
Supravalvular AS	I
7. Anomalies of the arteries	
Malpositions of the great arteries	II
Post-operative follow-up of shunts	I
Aortic (sinus of Valsalva) aneurysm	I
Aortic coarctation	I
Vascular rings	I
Patent ductus arteriosus	III
Aortopulmonary window	I
Coronary artery anomalies in infants	Inv
Anomalous origin of coronary arteries in adults and children	I
Pulmonary atresia	I
Central pulmonary stenosis	I
Peripheral pulmonary stenosis	Inv
Systemic to pulmonary collaterals	I

Table 1.8 Indications for CMR in acquired diseases of the vessels

Indication	Class
1. Diagnosis and follow-up of thoracic aortic aneurysm including Marfan disease	I
2. Diagnosis and planning of stent treatment for abdominal aortic aneurysm	II
3. Aortic dissection Diagnosis of acute aortic dissection Diagnosis and follow-up of chronic aortic dissection	II I
4. Diagnosis of aortic intramural haemorrhage	I
5. Diagnosis of penetrating ulcers of the aorta	I
6. PA anatomy and flow	I
7. Pulmonary emboli Diagnosis of central pulmonary emboli Diagnosis of peripheral pulmonary emboli	III Inv
8. Assessment of thoracic, abdominal and pelvic veins	I
9. Assessment of leg veins	II
10. Assessment of renal arteries	I
11. Assessment of mesenteric arteries	II
12. Assessment of iliac, femoral and lower leg arteries	I
13. Assessment of thoracic great vessel origins	I
14. Assessment of cervical carotid arteries	I
15. Assessment of atherosclerotic plaque in carotid artery/aorta	III
16. Assessment of pulmonary veins	I
17. Endothelial function	Inv

■ Contraindications and issues of safety

CMR is noninvasive and uses no ionizing radiation.

Contrast agents Gadolinium have very low nephrotoxicity but some agents have been linked to systematic fibrosis in renal failure.

Patients with prosthetic heart valves, sternal wires, joint replacements, retained epicardial pacing leads and intracoronary stents can be safely scanned.

CMR on patients with permanent pacemakers and automated implantable cardiac defibrillators (AICDs) should only be considered in specialist centres and remains a strong relative contraindication, while ferromagnetic cerebrovascular aneurysm clips are currently absolute contraindications.

There are no known risks for use during pregnancy, but CMR is usually avoided in the first trimester and used only for urgent clinical need after this time. Women who are breastfeeding must express and discard their breast milk for 24 hours after contrast use.

19

The environment in which CMR is performed must be constantly protected from the inadvertent introduction of ferromagnetic metallic objects and electronic equipment near the powerful magnetic field, with safety failures possibly leading to injury and rare cases of mortality. Potential subjects fill out a checklist as shown in Figure 1.10, which is then reviewed by trained personnel prior to placement within the magnet. Regular cardiorespiratory arrest scenario training in the safe and speedy removal of subjects undergoing CMR to nearby, designated resuscitation areas are advocated for clinical and allied MRI staff.

Checklist for subjects having a Cardiovascular Magnetic Resonance Scan

Name: Date of birth:

....

Hospital number: Height: Weight:

....

There are no known harmful effects of this scan but we need to know about any metallic objects or implants in the body, and some other conditions.

	Yes	No
Do you have a pacemaker or pacing wires in your heart?		
Do you have any other implants or metal in your body? e.g.: Hearing aid, ear or spine implant, programmable hydrocephalus shunt		
Have you had any operation on your head or spine?		
Have you had an injury to an eye which might have left metal in it?		
Have you had cardiac surgery?		
Do you have epilepsy, diabetes, asthma or allergies (if yes, please circle which)?		
Do you have a history of renal failure, or are you on dialysis?		
Are you wearing a nitro patch?		
Are you pregnant?		
Have you removed your watch, bankcards, spectacles, hearing aids, keys, coins, jewellery and hairgrips? (Gold rings are not a problem)		
	Please tick	

You may need to have an injection during the scan of a contrast agent or "dye" called gadolinium. This is a very safe procedure. At the time of the injection you may feel some sensations at the site of the injection and transient headache, nausea or a metallic taste can occur. Major side effects are very rare.

By signing below you acknowledge that the procedure has been explained to you by a qualified person, and that you have answered the above questions correctly.

Signature: ....   Witnessed by: ....

Date: ....

Figure 1.10 *Subjects are asked to fill in a safety questionnaire upon arrival for their CMR scan. The completed form is reviewed by trained personnel prior to commencement of the study. The questions are partly designed to identify contraindications to CMR, and partly to alert staff to important medical conditions which are not themselves contraindications.*

Chapter 2

Ischaemic heart disease

Katharina Kiss

■ Introduction

CMR is the current gold standard for the recognition of infarcted myocardium and the assessment of global and regional cardiac wall motion abnormalities (WMA). WMA arise in the context of MI and ischaemia. Stress-induced WMA are early indicators of coronary artery stenosis in the ischaemic cascade and may precede clinical symptoms and/or ECG changes (Figure 2.1). CMR can also diagnose haemodynamically significant coronary stenosis by measuring myocardial perfusion, although clinical experience is less extensive currently. Clinical CMR studies should follow the cardiac imaging protocol detailed in Chapter 1. Evaluation of global and regional ventricular function is by means of cines which reveal global and focal WMA. The four-chamber, two-chamber and short-axis stack cines are mandatory with subsequent imaging planes being directed by these initial views. These planes are repeated after gadolinium for imaging of myocardial pathology.

■ Myocardial infarction

Shortly after coronary artery occlusion, myocardial necrosis begins. This spreads outwards through the myocardial layers from the subendocardium towards the subepicardium. This progression of transmurality cannot be confidently discerned

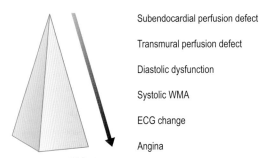

Subendocardial perfusion defect

Transmural perfusion defect

Diastolic dysfunction

Systolic WMA

ECG change

Angina

Figure 2.1 *The cascade of ischaemia shows that classic signs such as angina appear late in the course of ischaemic heart disease.*

with the ECG but is readily appreciated by CMR. Accurate imaging of infarcted territory is useful for diagnosis and in predicting outcomes such as the development of heart failure, and planning coronary arterial revascularization by either PCI (percutaneous coronary intervention) or CABG (coronary artery bypass grafting).

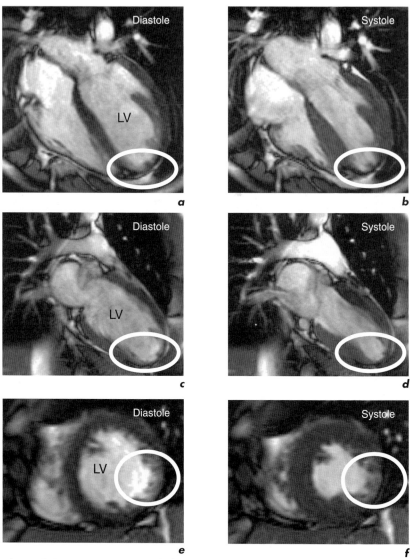

Figure 2.2 *Pre-contrast CMR study from a 26-year-old man who presented with dyspnoea, presyncope and palpitations. (**a, b**) Four-chamber view in diastole and systole. (**c, d**) Two-chamber view in diastole and systole. (**e, f**) Mid-ventricular short-axis view in diastole and systole. Comparison of these diastolic and systolic cine frames revealed global LV dilatation with thinning and akinesis in the lateral wall extending into the apex (white ellipses).*

Characteristic regional thinning of myocardium with akinesia suggests MI and is first noted on the cines (Figure 2.2). Exact delineation of damaged myocardium is then performed using the technique of late enhancement with gadolinium, or *LGE*.

Gadolinium is bound to a chelate in contrast agents which limits its distribution to the extracellular space. Gadolinium accumulates within abnormal interstitium in the myocardium affected by acute or chronic MI. In the acute setting gadolinium distributes into necrotic tissue, and in the chronic setting gadolinium is found in fibrosis of the infarct scar. Gadolinium accumulation reduces T1 and therefore increases signal on T1W images. This principle along with an ECG-gated, inversion recovery fast GE sequence underlies the LGE technique. An important additional feature of this technique is the inversion time delay set by the operator to optimize contrast between normal myocardium and infarcted tissue. With optimal setting of this inversion time, normal myocardium becomes black while infarcted myocardium is bright white. This has led to the aphorism that in infarction 'white is dead' (Figure 2.3).

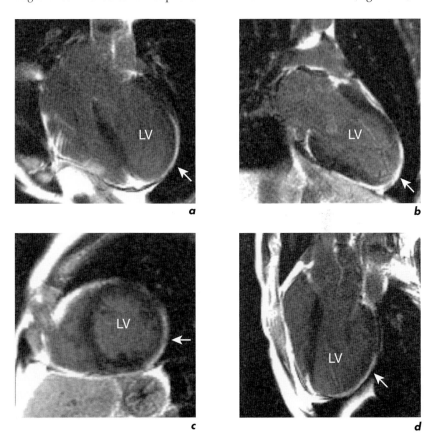

Figure 2.3 *LGE CMR study from the patient in Figure 2.2 which shows transmural enhancement within the left circumflex (LCx) territory (white arrows) in the **(a)** four-chamber, **(b)** two-chamber, **(c)** mid-ventricular short-axis and **(d)** LVOT views.*

CMR is also used to image zones of microvascular obstruction (MVO) using *early gadolinium enhancement (EGE)*. MVO occurs in the first hours post-MI, predicts an unfavourable prognosis, and corresponds to areas of no-reflow. The CMR appearances are of a black area within the infarct zone with exclusion of gadolinium relative to the surrounding reperfused infarcted tissue (Figure 2.4). These appearances also occur in LV thrombus and the clinical context of the CMR study must be borne in mind (Figure 2.5). EGE uses the same sequence as LGE but images are acquired in the

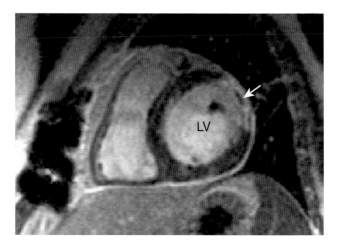

Figure 2.4 *Mid-ventricular short-axis view of an EGE study in an acute lateral MI showing a small dark zone of MVO embedded within the infarcted area (white arrow).*

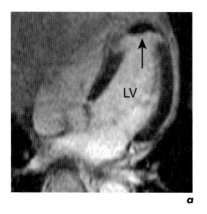
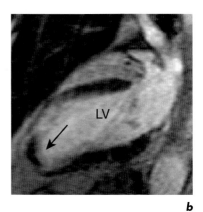

a

b

Figure 2.5 *(a) Four- and (b) two-chamber views from a 74-year-old man who had a history of MI in the left anterior descending artery (LAD) territory. EGE shows an LV apical thrombus (black arrows) overlying a transmural chronic infarct.*

first 1–5 minutes following contrast injection. LGE is commenced after 5 minutes have elapsed and imaging can continue for up to 20 minutes. The two-chamber, four-chamber and LVOT are standard views taken in EGE studies. For LGE a full short-axis stack and long-axis images are acquired. Additional imaging through areas of known or suspected pathology are recommended and positive findings are reported as *early* or *late enhancement*, respectively.

The technique takes approximately 20 minutes to perform and begins with dose calculation of gadolinium, selection of initial views, and setting of the inversion time. Images are acquired in late diastole when cardiac motion artefact should be minimal. Another artefact reduction technique is the application of a saturation prepulse over the spinal column to overcome the problem of cerebrospinal fluid (CSF) ghosting (Figure 2.6). Gadolinium is typically given at a dose of 0.1 mmol/kg by rapid hand injection into a peripheral vein. Inversion time for EGE imaging is set at 440 milliseconds (ms) and reduced to around 320 ms for LGE imaging to commence. Throughout the LGE acquisition, the inversion time is gradually increased up to 440 ms to maintain correct signal nulling of normal myocardium (Figure 2.7). Abnormal findings should be confirmed by changing the phase encode direction of the slice to confidently exclude artefact (Figure 2.8). This is known as *phase-swapping*.

So in the setting of MI, CMR can:

1. Evaluate global and regional cardiac function;
2. Demonstrate wall thickness and contractility; and
3. Highlight zones of MVO (or thrombus) and transmurality of infarction with EGE and LGE.

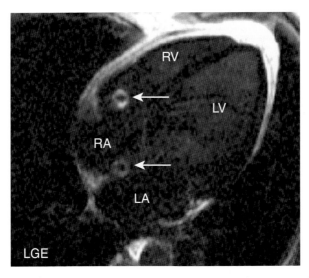

Figure 2.6 Four-chamber LGE image showing CSF ghosting (white arrows) along the phase encode axis.

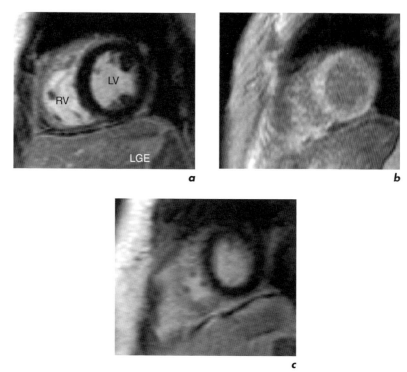

Figure 2.7 LGE mid-ventricular short-axis views of the appearance of the myocardium when the inversion time is set **(a)** too short, **(b)** too long and **(c)** correctly.

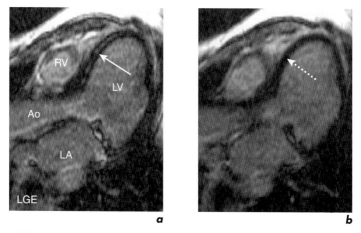

Figure 2.8 LVOT view showing artefactual late enhancement within the interventricular septum (IVS) **(a**; solid white arrow), which disappears upon changing the direction of the phase encode axis **(b**; dashed white arrow).

The scan report should address all these issues and will be discussed in more detail in the next section on myocardial viability.

■ Myocardial viability

Viable myocardium exhibits contractile dysfunction at baseline but recovery over time either spontaneously after MI (myocardial stunning) or after physical re-establishment of coronary blood flow (hibernating myocardium). CMR can differentiate between viable myocardium and areas of infarction using LGE since, in the former, significant WMA are present but late enhancement is absent or limited. Combination of CMR findings and clinical history allows further discrimination.

Stunned myocardium is usually a transient phenomenon seen after ischaemia often in the setting of an occluded coronary artery. With chronically impaired maximal myocardial perfusion, such as in the presence of a severe coronary artery stenosis, hibernation may occur with chronic WMA. Patients with hibernating myocardium tend to have multivessel disease and impaired LV function. Regional WMA can persist for six months or longer after successful revascularization of hibernation without evidence of myocardial necrosis according to the severity of the baseline myocardial cellular derangement.

CMR assessment of viability is performed as discussed in section 2.1 on MI with cine imaging and LGE. The cine slices and equivalent LGE views must be reviewed in parallel to correlate the following parameters:

1. Wall thickness and contractility;
2. Presence or absence of WMA; both with respect to
3. Presence or absence of LGE and degree of transmurality.

For example, significant wall thinning and impaired contractility in association with akinesia and transmural late enhancement indicates myocardial scarring. However, reduced contractility in association with normal thickness and no late enhancement indicates viable hibernating myocardium (Figure 2.9). This mismatch between cines and contrast findings is the key to reporting myocardial viability CMR studies. LGE CMR can quantify the degree of transmural involvement in MI and as transmurality increases the likelihood of improvement in regional contractility post-revascularization decreases.

> Dysfunctional myocardium which shows < 50% transmural gadolinium enhancement has a high likelihood of functional recovery (Figure 2.10), while transmural infarction of > 75% is unlikely to recover contractility (Figure 2.3).

The scan report should follow the 17-segment model (Figure 2.11) and include:

1. Qualitative and quantitative description of global and regional ventricular function;
2. A description of the severity of WMA and percentage of transmural LGE following the 17-segment model; and
3. Correlation of these two parameters to indicate which segments are viable.

Persistent WMA post-MI with successful revascularization may reflect delayed recovery and warrants repeat CMR evaluation after 4–6 months. Perfusion CMR or a dobutamine stress CMR can further clarify the issue of stunned versus hibernating myocardium.

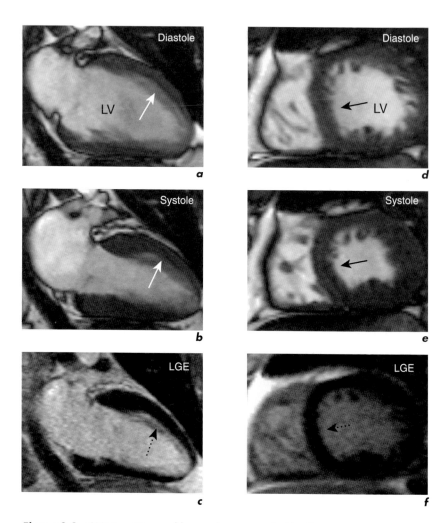

Figure 2.9 *CMR in a 51-year-old man who presented with a Troponin positive acute coronary syndrome. X-ray coronary angiography had previously revealed a 50% stenosis in the LAD. **(a, b)** Two-chamber view in diastole and systole with the equivalent slice after gadolinium in **(c)**. **(d, e)** Mid-ventricular short-axis view in diastole and systole with the equivalent slice after gadolinium in **(f)**. These images demonstrate wall thinning and reduced contractility in the distal anterior wall (solid white arrows) and septum (solid black arrows) which were associated with WMA but no late enhancement (dashed black arrows) and good biventricular function. Such findings indicate myocardial stunning.*

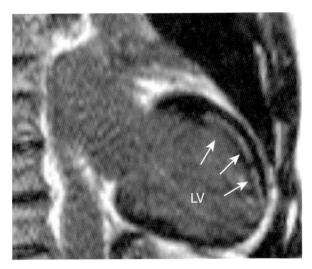

Figure 2.10 *Two-chamber view showing non-transmural LGE in the anterior wall (white arrows) indicating subendocardial anterior MI.*

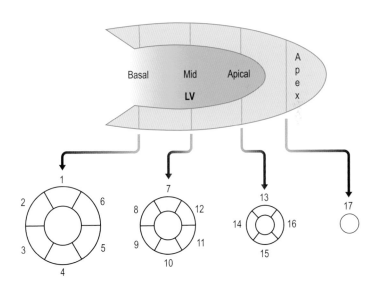

Figure 2.11 *Modified schematic of the 17-segment model proposed by the American Heart Association for describing area of LV involvement:*
1 = basal anterior, 2 = basal anteroseptal, 3 = basal inferoseptal, 4 = basal inferior, 5 = basal inferolateral, 6 = basal anterolateral; 7 = mid-anterior, 8 = mid-anteroseptal, 9 = mid-inferoseptal, 10 = mid-inferior, 11 = mid-inferolateral, 12 = mid-anterolateral; 13 = apical anterior, 14 = apical septal, 15 = apical inferior, 16 = apical lateral, 17 = apex.

■ Myocardial perfusion

Resting coronary blood flow increases with exercise or other stress. This increase in coronary blood flow is the coronary flow reserve ($Flow_{stress} / Flow_{rest} = CFR$) with a normal range of approximately 4. With significant stenosis, coronary blood flow cannot increase adequately with stress and an inducible perfusion defect becomes apparent in the relevant coronary artery territory (Figure 2.12). Perfusion CMR can identify this perfusion defect and there is good correlation with myocardial scintigraphy. However, compared to scintigraphy, CMR allows improved resolution with no ionizing radiation. The optimal imaging sequence for perfusion CMR is currently multislice, single-shot hybrid GE using imaging acceleration during the first pass of a bolus of gadolinium. Good temporal (approximately 50–100 ms/image with certain sequences) and spatial resolution (approximately 2–3 mm) is essential in eliminating subendocardial artefacts which can mimic perfusion defects.

Pharmacological stress is usually with adenosine and contraindications are those of the CMR itself or for use of this agent. Caution is required in patients with unstable angina, stenotic valvular disease, reversible obstructive lung disease and sino-atrial disease. Patients must omit caffeine-containing products (such as coffee, tea and chocolate) for 24 hours beforehand as these are adenosine antagonists. Continuous ECG and blood pressure monitoring is mandatory.

A perfusion CMR study incorporates functional and LGE evaluation and takes approximately 45 minutes to perform. Standard planes are obtained as described in the pre-contrast section outlined in Table 1.1. It is important to position the basal short-axis so as to avoid the LVOT throughout the cardiac cycle for avoidance of misinterpretation of abnormalities from the fibrous septum. The stress part of the perfusion examination is then performed during an infusion of intravenous adenosine (140 μg/kg/min for 4 minutes into the left antecubital vein) with a bolus of intravenous Gd-DTPA (0.1 mmol/kg at a rate of 7 ml/s followed by 15 ml of normal saline at the same rate via a large bore cannula in the right antecubital vein) given after 2 minutes and at the commencement of the perfusion sequence. Typically three ventricular short-axis slices are acquired in a breath-hold at end-expiration over the first cardiac cycles of the first pass. Image acquisition is over 60 seconds and patients are instructed to breathe gently when needed. Rest perfusion is delayed for 20 minutes after stress perfusion in order to reduce gadolinium levels, and is performed using the same doses and rates of gadolinium and saline as those for stress but without the adenosine.

The perfusion CMR scan report should follow the 17-segment model (Figure 2.11) and include:

1. Anatomical description of the perfusion defects;
2. Correlation of these defects with the pattern and percentage of LGE;
3. Description of viability; and
4. Quantitation of ventricular function.

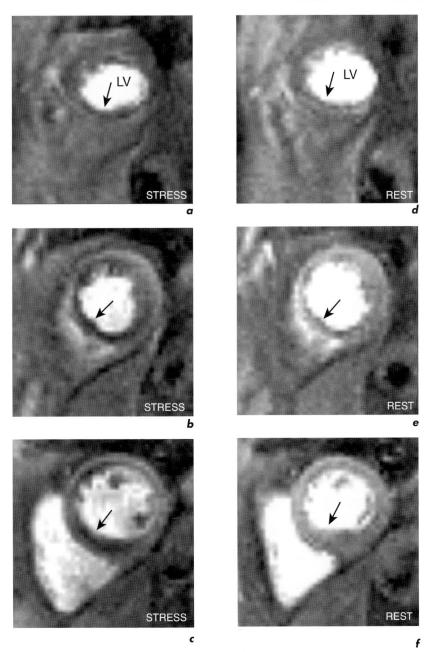

Figure 2.12 Perfusion CMR in three ventricular short-axis views during adenosine stress **(a–c)** and rest **(d–f)** in a 58-year-old man prior to CABG showing inducible ischaemia of the inferoseptal wall in the territory of the right coronary artery (RCA) (black arrows).

■ Dobutamine stress testing

Viable myocardium that is hibernating will often improve contractility during stress. Pharmacological stress is usually with the catecholamine dobutamine which acts at cardiac β_1 receptors to increase myocardial oxygen demand. Patients should avoid beta-blockers for 24 hours prior to the scan. Continuous ECG monitoring with pulse oximetry and blood pressure measurements every minute are required, along with direct questioning of patients during the study regarding adverse events. Side effects include nausea, dizziness, dyspnoea, chest pain and palpitations, and serious adverse events include induction of ventricular arrhythmias or prolonged ischaemia.

Two protocols are available—a low-dose dobutamine protocol using 10μg/kg/min administered to assess viability, and a high-dose dobutamine protocol using up to 40μg/kg/min to detect ischaemia. During low-dose protocols, the focus is on the improvement of WMA present at rest in order to differentiate between viable and non-viable myocardium. The high-dose protocol is similar to dobutamine stress echocardiography (DSE). Two- and four-chamber views with representative ventricular short-axis slices are used. The initial dose with both protocols is 5μg/kg/min. This is increased to 10μg/kg/min after 3 minutes. With high-dose dobutamine stress, doses are increased every 4 minutes by 10μg/kg/min with constant monitoring for WMA. Dobutamine stress studies are usually terminated when the target heart rate is achieved (target heart rate = 0.85 [220 − age]) or after peak dobutamine dose. If the patient has a poor heart rate response to dobutamine, atropine can be given in small repeated doses.

A dobutamine stress CMR examination takes 45 minutes to perform. Data analysis and reporting should follow the 17-segment model (Figure 2.11) and provide information on:

1. Resting regional WMA and EF; and
2. Improvements in contractility or identification of new WMA with stress.

■ Indications

CMR can:

1. Offer superior image quality to echocardiography for the detection of WMA;
2. Provide the gold standard for quantification and reproducibility of LV and RV function;
3. Demonstrate MVO and transmurality of MI and therefore predict the likelihood of wall motion recovery after revascularization; and
4. Provide high-resolution myocardial perfusion imaging without ionizing radiation.

CMR cannot:

1. Be recommended for quantification of stenoses within native coronary arteries. Coronary magnetic resonance angiography (MRA) has an 81% negative predictive value for the exclusion of multivessel proximal CAD.

Assessment of bypass graft patency is straightforward using CMR, but computed tomography (CT) is more commonly used. Coronary MRA is reliable for identification of coronary artery anomalies.

Chapter 3

Heart failure and cardiomyopathy

James C Moon

■ Introduction

Heart failure is a complex syndrome in which the heart functions inadequately as a pump to support a physiological circulation resulting in symptoms such as breathlessness and fatigue and signs such as fluid retention. It is associated with high morbidity and mortality and represents a major burden for healthcare services.

The aetiology of heart failure includes CAD, hypertension, valvular pathology, and much rarer inherited heart muscle diseases. Additionally, conditions such as pulmonary or renal disease can mimic the symptoms and signs. The management of heart failure rests upon accurate diagnosis and elucidation of the underlying aetiology. This requires thorough clinical evaluation and appropriately targeted investigations. ECG and echocardiography are the usual initial investigations and CMR is a complementary tool that can provide important quantitative and qualitative insights, especially with regard to the cardiomyopathies.

The cardiomyopathies are diseases of the myocardium associated with cardiac dysfunction and are subdivided on the basis of morphology into hypertrophic, dilated, restrictive and ARVC (Figure 3.1). Many cardiomyopathies are inherited through a single gene abnormality. Some cardiomyopathies have an extended phenotype with conduction disease, whilst other genetic cardiac diseases have conduction disease (such as long/short QT and the Brugada syndrome—the channelopathies) without 'cardiomyopathy'. At least nine different sarcomeric genes can cause the same phenotype of hypertrophic cardiomyopathy (HCM) and yet different mutations in some of these nine genes can also cause DCM. Approximately half of all HCM patients have been shown to have a genetic mutation and many individuals carry mutations without phenotypic manifestation, and the impact of environment, genetic modifiers and patient age are important. There are also disease mimics known as *phenocopies*, such as the glycogen storage diseases, which appear phenotypically like the genetic diseases.

CMR is the best single technique for defining the cardiomyopathy phenotype, detecting early phenotypic changes, defining aetiology and distinguishing phenocopies, assessing response to treatment, and potentially aiding risk stratification.

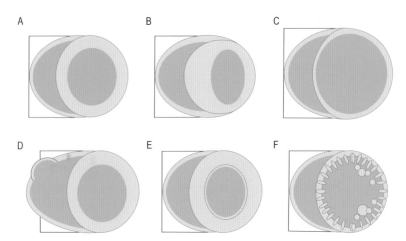

Figure 3.1 *Classification of cardiomyopathies by morphology.*
(a) Normal; *(b)* hypertrophic; *(c)* dilated; *(d)* arrhythmogenic right ventricular;
(e) restrictive—the endocardial lines represent dysfunctional long-axis fibres; *(f)* non-compaction—the endocardium has an open trabecular structure with relative thinning of the compacted myocardium.

■ CMR protocol

A CMR heart failure and cardiomyopathy protocol typically obtains information on cardiac morphology, cardiac function and myocardial tissue characterization. The scan report should comment on these three areas in general terms such as:

1. Cardiac chamber size;
2. Quantitative values for cardiac function and mass with respect to the reference ranges quoted in Chapter 1; and
3. The presence (with a description of the pattern) or absence of LGE.

Specific features for reporting are highlighted after discussion of the specific cardiomyopathies.

Cardiac morphology

The anatomical structure of the heart can be shown using different types of sequences and the white-blood and black-blood techniques previously described provide complementary information. For example, black-blood imaging is extensively used for imaging the RV in ARVC, while white-blood SSFP cines best define left ventricular non-compaction (LVNC).

Cardiac function

CMR is the gold standard technique for the assessment of left and right ventricular volumes and mass due to a combination of advantages (Table 3.1). CMR measurements

Table 3.1 Advantages of CMR for measuring ventricular function

Precise and reproducible piloting
No problems with acoustic windows
No blind spots—image quality the same throughout
High blood–myocardial tissue contrast (even in heart failure)
True 3D assessment with no geometric assumptions
RV imaged as well as the LV
Any view or plane can be imaged as necessary

are more reproducible than echocardiography, the apex and RV are no longer blind spots (Figure 3.2), and the technique is not window dependent (Figure 3.3). For heart failure, the SSFP GE cine sequences have major advantages because the blood to myocardium contrast is dependent not on blood flow but on intrinsic magnetic differences between blood and myocardium. This means that the blood pool is more clearly distinguished from myocardium even in slow-flow areas compared to that using older white-blood imaging methods. The SSFP sequences can also be sped up using parallel imaging acquisition techniques to minimize breath-holding times in symptomatic heart failure patients.

An emerging technique for functional assessment is *myocardial tagging*. In this technique, a grid of tag lines is laid over the heart magnetically in diastole and then tracked as they distort with myocardial contraction through systole (Figure 3.4). The tag line deformation can be analysed like tissue Doppler imaging, but rather

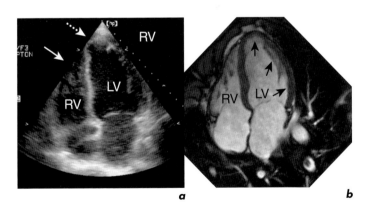

a *b*

Figure 3.2 *Four-chamber views comparing (a) a transthoracic echocardiogram (TTE) and (b) a CMR still of a cine loop in the same individual. CMR displays the RV (solid white arrow), apex (dashed white arrow), and endocardial border (solid black arrows) more clearly.*

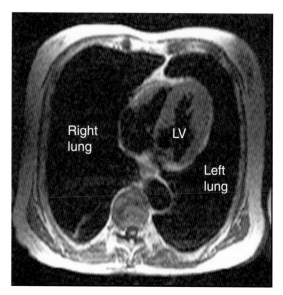

Figure 3.3 *A pilot transaxial FSE CMR image from a patient with emphysema in whom the TTE provided poor acoustic windows.*

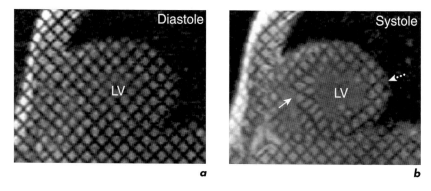

Figure 3.4 *Myocardial tagging of a mid-ventricular short-axis slice in **(a)** diastole and **(b)** systole following an acute MI. The grid of tag lines is laid down in diastole and cardiac motion results in distortion (strain and torsion) in systole. The septum shows normal contractile function (short white arrow), but the lateral wall tag lines are unchanged (dashed white arrow), highlighting contractile dysfunction within this area.*

than being limited to strain in line with the Doppler beam, tagging can be analysed in any direction simultaneously, including circumferentially, at any point in the myocardium, and is able to compare epicardial and endocardial function.

Myocardial tissue characterization

Normal and abnormal myocardium can have *intrinsic contrast* differences in heart failure that can be visualized by CMR. For example, fatty infiltration of the RV may be seen in ARVC using FSE sequences with and without the addition of a specially applied fat saturation pulse, which eliminates only fat from the images. Also, tissues which have increased water content, such as in myocardial oedema from acute infiltration or infarction, can be differentiated with T2W sequences (Figure 3.5). *Extrinsic contrast* can be created by LGE, which uses an inversion recovery sequence and a gadolinium contrast agent (see Chapter 2). Gadolinium highlights areas of myocardium with expanded interstitium, such as fibrosis, necrosis or infiltration. Different patterns of fibrosis exist in different aetiologies of heart failure and this can be used to distinguish them (Figure 3.6). MI leads to patterns of LGE which spread from the subendocardium outward to the subepicardium in the territory of a coronary artery. However, changes in myocarditis are the reverse and start at the subepicardium and can later become mid-myocardial, typically at the lateral wall. EGE in combination with relevant cines allows identification of thrombi. This technique has been discussed in the previous chapter and will also be covered in Chapter 5 on cardiac masses. Coronary CMR assessment of the proximal coronary arterial tree can be combined with myocardial tissue characterization but this technique is not robust—it is further discussed in Chapter 9.

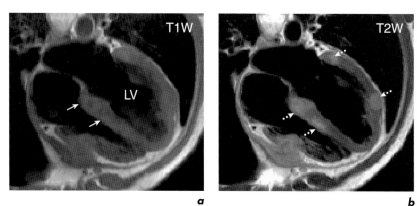

a *b*

Figure 3.5 **(a)** T1W and **(b)** T2W four-chamber views in a case of myocardial lymphoma showing interventricular septal infiltration. The septum is distorted by infiltration on the T1W image, but appears similar in contrast to normal myocardium (solid white arrows). However, subsequent T2W imaging shows high signal indicative of oedema in both the septum and the lateral wall (dashed white arrows).

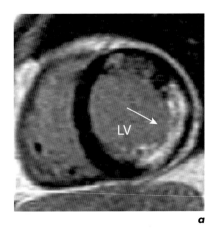 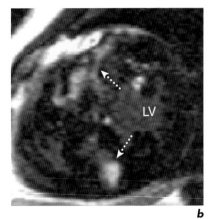

a   *b*

Figure 3.6 *Myocardium infarcted or fibrotic appears bright with LGE. The characteristic pattern of subendocardial enhancement in a coronary artery territory is shown post-MI (**a**; solid white arrow) as distinct from the pattern of contrast uptake noted with focal fibrosis in HCM (**b**; dashed white arrows).*

■ CMR in selected cardiomyopathies

Hypertrophic cardiomyopathy

HCM strictly includes the sarcomeric variants but the phenocopies are also discussed here since the differentiation of these two groups is an important role of CMR (Table 3.2). The HCM phenotype shows high variability and also changes throughout

Table 3.2   Phenocopies of sarcomeric HCM
Storage diseases
Anderson–Fabry disease
Glycogen storage diseases
Mucopolysaccharidoses
Mitochondrial myopathies
Syndromes (Noonan's, Friedreich's ataxia)
Physiological hypertrophy
Increased afterload (hypertension, AS, outflow tract obstruction)
Athlete's heart
Afro-Caribbean
Compensatory hypertrophy (after MI)
Infiltration
Amyloid
Senile amyloid
Ageing
Sigmoid septum

life. Expression of early familial disease may be with an abnormal ECG and normal echocardiogram, fulfilling proposed familial criteria for HCM. In a proportion of these, CMR can detect early hypertrophy overlooked at echocardiography. CMR is especially useful in disease which is limited to the LV apex (Figure 3.7). Indicators of apical HCM in the context of non-diagnostic echocardiography include giant negative T waves on the ECG and subtle echocardiographic abnormalities such as diastolic dysfunction and apical akinesis.

In established HCM, there is a need to identify patients at risk of sudden death and this is mainly done by assessing the presence of known risk factors such as family history of sudden death, unexplained syncope, ventricular tachycardia, abnormal exercise test, and LV wall thickness greater than 30 mm. Adding up the number of risk factors gives a reasonable indication of risk. In the absence of any risk factors, the patient is considered low risk and management is with reassurance and regular reassessment. In the presence of more than two risk factors, patients are high risk and warrant anti-arrhythmia treatment, often with an AICD. However, a third of patients have only one risk factor and are at intermediate risk. LGE CMR may help further risk stratify this group into low or high risk since myocardial fibrosis may represent the substrate for heart failure and arrhythmias (Figure 3.8). The risk of sudden death is greater in those with greater myocardial late enhancement and in the presence of progressive LV dilatation and thinning. This is especially true for the younger patient population (< 40 years old). The specific pattern of LGE may also be important and is also helpful in distinguishing HCM mimics such as Anderson–Fabry disease (AFD). AFD is an X-linked storage disease that causes left ventricular hypertrophy (LVH) and accounts for 1 to 3% of patients with phenotypic HCM. AFD should be considered in middle-aged men with suspected HCM where an auto-somal dominant family history is not present, especially if there is no evidence of

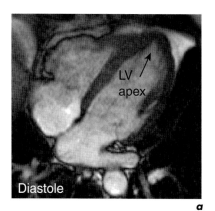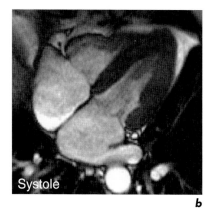

a *b*

Figure 3.7 *Four-chamber SSFP cine CMR images from a 51-year-old man referred with an abnormal resting ECG but normal TTE and X-ray coronary angiography. There is **(a)** hypertrophy at the LV apex in diastole associated with **(b)** LV cavity obliteration in systole, indicating a diagnosis of apical HCM.*

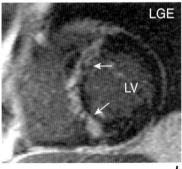

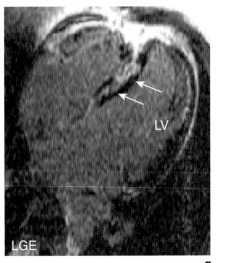

Figure 3.8 *Post-contrast CMR study from a 43-year-old man with a strong family history of HCM, mildly decreased LV function on TTE, and normal coronary arteries. The **(a)** four-chamber and **(b)** mid-ventricular short-axis views show extensive late enhancement of the interventricular septum (white arrows), which is not subendocardial as with MI.*

LVOT obstruction. Contrast enhancement in AFD occurs predominantly at the basal inferolateral wall. Other mimics include cardiac amyloid where the heart is infiltrated with the amyloid protein. This protein accumulates preferentially throughout the subendocardium, the site of the longitudinal fibres, leading to reduced long-axis function. The myocardium becomes non-compliant and exhibits a restrictive physiology. There is symmetrical and global myocardial hypertrophy, which is readily visualized by CMR, and there may be characteristic subendocardial contrast enhancement and a black-blood pool due to rapid wash-out of gadolinium from the blood (Figure 3.9).

Up to a quarter of patients with HCM have LVOT obstruction. In LVOT obstruction, the AMVL or papillary muscles move forward into the outflow tract in systole where they flutter and may hinder the ejection of blood. This may be associated with a posteriorly directed jet of mitral regurgitation (MR). Treatment is mainly with beta-blockers but surgical myomectomy or alcohol ablation can be performed. Alcohol ablation involves injection of alcohol into the first septal artery causing infarction of the myocardium in that territory and relieving the obstruction. Subsequent scar formation and remodelling can be evaluated using CMR. Rarely, a residual ridge of myocardium remains which causes further obstruction and can be evaluated at follow-up CMR.

Specific features for reporting on are:

1. Measurements of differential septal thickness (asymmetric septal hypertrophy);
2. LVOT obstruction or systolic anterior motion of the AMVL;

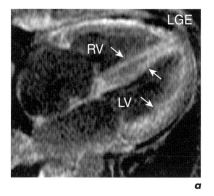
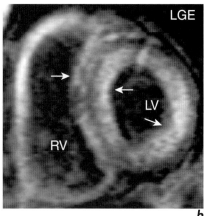

Figure 3.9 **(a)** *Four-chamber and* **(b)** *mid-ventricular short-axis views of global late enhancement which spares the subepicardium that is characteristic of cardiac amyloid (white arrows). Late enhancement in this setting is due to amyloid protein deposition as opposed to myocardial fibrosis.*

3. Comments on function, morphology, and presence (and pattern) of LGE and changes since preceding studies.

Dilated cardiomyopathy

CMR evaluation of DCM has several components. Early LV dilatation is quantified volumetrically and can be compared with age, gender and body surface area normalized reference ranges. The size of the heart in relation to the chest is also immediately apparent.

> CMR can distinguish DCM from cardiac chamber dilatation due to CAD using LGE, and this may obviate the need for cardiac catheterization in some patients.

When cardiac dilatation heart due to coronary disease is advanced, myocardial wall thinning due to infarction, remote remodelling and subendocardial infarction can make the appearance of the heart very similar to that found in DCM. LGE CMR studies in this situation demonstrate transmural or subendocardial MI. By contrast, in most cases of DCM there is either no enhancement or a characteristic mid-myocardial wall fibrosis affecting the circumferential fibres (Figure 3.10). Late enhancement in some suspected cases of DCM may represent sequelae of previous myocarditis.

Specific comments for the CMR report in DCM are:

1. Quantification of normalized biventricular function;
2. Evidence of DCM as opposed to coronary disease; and
3. Changes in function, morphology and contrast enhancement since previous imaging.

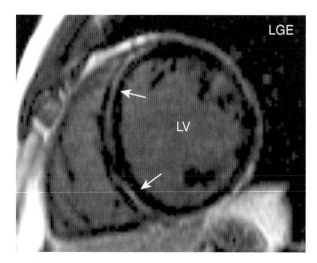

Figure 3.10 *Mid-ventricular short-axis view post-contrast demonstrating the characteristic mid-myocardial wall late enhancement seen in DCM (white arrows).*

Thalassaemia major

Thalassaemia is a common genetic condition worldwide which results in anaemia secondary to defective globin synthesis. β-Thalassaemia major is the homozygous form of defective β-globin synthesis and affected individuals are blood transfusion dependent. Repeated transfusions contribute to iron overload and iron becomes deposited throughout the body, especially the heart, liver, pancreas and endocrine glands. The resulting cardiomyopathy can progress to overt cardiac failure which can be rapidly progressive. Mortality in thalassaemia major is often from heart failure, with many patients dying prematurely in their mid-thirties. Timely detection of cardiac dysfunction allows targeting of aggressive iron chelation therapy in these individuals and can reverse the cardiomyopathic process.

Currently, no echocardiographic criteria have been established for the pre-clinical diagnosis of iron overload cardiomyopathy and haematologists have therefore relied upon serum ferritin measurements and liver biopsy findings to act as surrogates for quantification of cardiac iron burden. Serum ferritin is influenced by many factors and cannot specify the organ affected and iron deposition within the liver is poorly correlated to cardiac iron loading.

Actual myocardial iron concentration can be more directly and better quantified using a multiecho T2* GE CMR technique which measures the myocardial relaxation parameter known as 'T2 star' (Figure 3.11). Myocardial T2* measurements are made using a mid-ventricular short-axis slice and normal values are approximately 40 ms, with a lower boundary of 20 ms. In thalassaemia, values greater than 20 ms suggest no significant iron loading whilst values less than 10 ms indicate severe iron loading (Table 3.3). Approximately 90% of patients presenting in heart failure have

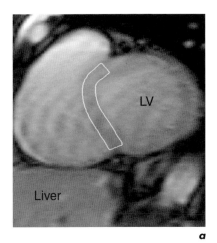

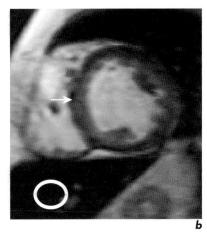

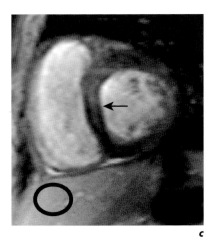

Figure 3.11 *The T2* GE CMR technique for measurement of cardiac iron status.*
(a) CMR appearance in a normal subject. T2* measurements are made in a mid-ventricular short-axis view within the area of IVS as highlighted. (b) Example of iron deposition in a patient with thalassaemia major. The IVS now has a dark epicardial rim indicating significant cardiac iron loading (white arrow). Iron deposition within the liver is also heavy and the liver therefore appears black (white ellipse). This signal loss occurs because of disturbances in the relaxation parameters of the tissues brought about by the iron causing alterations in the local magnetic field. (c) Another case of thalassaemia major which highlights the poor correlation between iron deposition in the heart (black arrow) and the liver (black ellipse). This means that optimal management of myocardial iron overload to prevent cardiac complications (arrhythmia, heart failure and death) in these patients cannot be conducted via the surrogate marker of liver iron content.

Table 3.3 Guidelines for iron assessment

Iron loading	Myocardial T2* (ms)	Hepatic T2* (ms)
None	> 20	> 6.3
Mild	14–20	2.7–6.3
Moderate	10–14	1.4–2.7
Severe	< 10	< 1.4

a T2* of less than 10 ms and are at high risk of death. They require urgent increases of iron chelation therapy, often with two drugs. Liver T2* measurements are made in a hepatic transaxial slice avoiding hepatic blood vessels. Values greater than 6.3 ms indicate no significant iron loading and values less than 1.4 ms indicate severe iron loading (Table 3.3). The total study duration is approximately 15 minutes and the technique can also be used in other iron overload conditions such as haemochromatosis and sickle cell anaemia.

Specific elements of the CMR report are:

1. Myocardial T2* quantification;
2. Hepatic T2* quantification; and
3. Comments on changes in cardiac function and T2* parameters since previous studies.

Arrhythmogenic right ventricular cardiomyopathy

In ARVC, ventricular tachycardia arising from the RV may cause sudden death. The disease is usually autosomal dominant with abnormalities in genes coding for proteins in the cell junctions known as desmosomes. Injury results from impaired tissue integrity with fibro-fatty healing typically affecting the thinner walled RV. Affected individuals can have associated abnormalities of RV and LV structure, and the former are better delineated by CMR than TTE (Figure 3.12). Abnormalities include regional RV WMA, wall thinning, fatty infiltration and LGE. In the late stages, the RV may become poorly functioning. Early changes are difficult to detect and there are traps for the unwary: in the normal RV, the free wall at the moderator insertion may appear akinetic, normal RV wall motion is highly variable, and intra-myocardial fat must be distinguished from epicardial fat. CMR in ARVC requires experience, results must be interpreted in conjunction with the defined major and minor criteria and with other clinical tests to generate an overall probability of disease.

The specific CMR comments here reflect the underlying suspected or known diagnosis:

1. Quantification of biventricular function;
2. Evidence of WMA or aneurysmal changes, especially of the RV free wall, apex and RVOT;
3. Evidence of fatty infiltration or LGE.

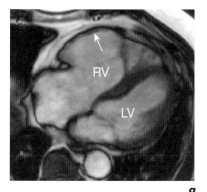

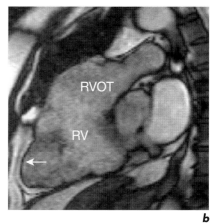

a

b

Figure 3.12   *CMR in a patient with ARVC referred with intermittent broad complex tachycardia maintained on amiodarone. The RV had already been noted as abnormal on TTE. **(a)** Four-chamber cine CMR showing localized aneurysmal section of the RV free wall (white arrow) which was dyskinetic. **(b)** RVOT cine CMR showing thinning of the RV. The aneurysmal area is once again noted (white arrow) and there is associated dilatation of the RV and RVOT (≥ LVOT diameter).*

Other cardiomyopathies

Restrictive cardiomyopathies are well visualized with CMR and key features include reduced long-axis function and atrial dilatation. In addition, subendocardial enhancement may be seen. Examples of diseases that cause a restrictive pattern include cardiac amyloid (Figure 3.9) and eosinophilic heart disease causing endomyocardial fibrosis.

Cardiac sarcoid can also cause fibrosis, visible by LGE, often with dense punched-out lesions. Myocardial oedema may be present on T2W images in association with active inflammation.

LVNC is a cardiomyopathy characterized by an altered structure of the LV myocardium with very thinned, hypokinetic segments consisting of two layers: thin, compacted myocardium on the subepicardial side, and a thicker non-compacted subendocardial layer (Figure 3.13). RV non-compaction accompanies LVNC in a significant proportion of patients. Clinical manifestations include heart failure, ventricular arrhythmias and systemic embolic events. TTE and CMR are the imaging methods of choice with the criteria for diagnosis being a ratio of non-compacted to compacted myocardial layers of greater than 2.

■ Indications

CMR can:

1. Determine LV and RV cardiac morphology and function normalized to sex, age and body surface area;
2. Reproducibly assess cardiac function and so accurately monitor response to drug therapy;

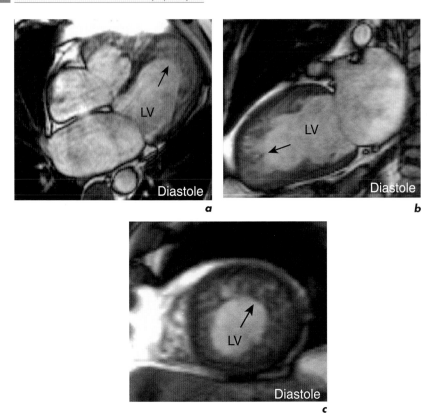

Figure 3.13 *(a) Four-chamber, (b) two-chamber and (c) mid-ventricular short-axis SSFP cine CMR images from a 68-year-old man with known LVNC highlighting the pathognomonic combination of multiple prominent ventricular trabeculations and deep intertrabecular recesses in communication with the ventricular cavity (black arrows).*

3. Detect myocardial oedema/iron/fat;
4. Visualize myocardial fibrosis and protein deposition;
5. Differentiate between DCM and cardiac dilatation due to CAD; and
6. Distinguish between the cardiomyopathies (assign the phenotype).

CMR cannot:

1. Replace comprehensive multimodality assessment—history taking, clinical examination, chest X-ray, ECG and echocardiography;
2. Diagnose channelopathies/ARVC in the structurally normal heart;
3. Detect short temporal resolution events (premature valve opening/closure, isovolumetric times, subtle dyssynchrony);
4. Quantify diastolic dysfunction with the temporal resolution of echocardiography; and
5. Image patients after device therapy (MRI-compatible pacemakers are currently being evaluated).

Chapter 4

Valvular heart disease

George E Gentchos and Marc D Tischler

■ Introduction

Cine imaging using SSFP and velocity mapping sequences are the cornerstone of CMR valvular assessment. Breath-hold high-resolution FSE can be useful for valve morphology and developments such as moving slice velocity mapping and real-time imaging will improve evaluation in the near future. CMR reporting in valvular heart disease generally includes:

1. Comments on cardiac chamber size;
2. Quantitative values for cardiac function and mass with respect to the reference ranges quoted in Chapter 1; and
3. Details of valve morphology where possible.

Further reporting requirements are highlighted following discussion of the specific valvular lesions.

■ Aortic stenosis

AS can occur at the valvular, subvalvular or supravalvular level. Valvular AS most commonly occurs with degeneration of a normal three-cusp aortic valve architecture. Bicuspid valves degenerate far earlier than tricuspid valves and are the second most common cause of AS in the adult, with rheumatic heart disease being the third. Subvalvular AS is caused by a fibrous or fibromuscular membrane which encircles the LVOT causing outflow tract obstruction. These patients typically present in adulthood with recurrence of a previously resected subvalvular membrane. Subvalvular stenosis can also be caused by asymmetric septal hypertrophy, abnormal MV or papillary muscle insertion, or posterior displacement of the infundibular septum. Supravalvular AS is uncommon, producing narrowing usually at the sino-tubular junction. It occurs in patients with Williams syndrome (60%), and there are familial forms and sporadic idiopathic cases.

AS has a long asymptomatic period after which clinical symptoms such as angina, exertional dyspnoea and effort syncope may result. Since symptoms develop late in the pathophysiology of AS, clinical deterioration soon follows if valve replacement is not undertaken. Obstruction to the LVOT leads to elevated LV pressures and compensatory LVH which initially maintains cardiac output and reduces LV wall stress, but ultimately decreases LV compliance and increases end-diastolic pressure. Increased myocardial oxygen demand causes myocardial ischaemia and later LV failure.

CMR is a robust method of calculating the severity of AS and correlates well with continuous wave Doppler echocardiography. However, it is far superior to echocardiography in identifying the cardiovascular functional and morphological sequelae of AS, such as post-stenotic dilatation of the ascending aorta, degree of LVH, and myocardial viability (Figures 4.1 and 4.2). These are important factors in

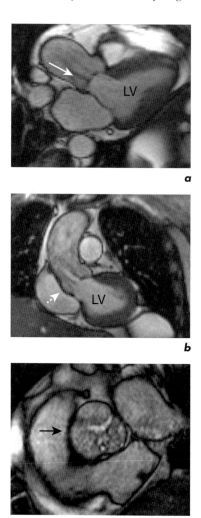

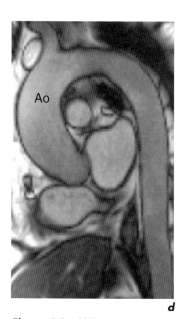

Figure 4.1 *SSFP cine images illustrating part of the CMR assessment in a 66-year-old man with mild AS. The first LVOT view (**a**) shows signal loss across the AV indicative of turbulent blood flow (solid white arrow) and no evidence of LVH. The second LVOT view (**b**) reveals mild aortic root dilatation at the sinuses of Valsalva (dashed white arrow). The AV is trileaflet (**c**; black arrow) and the remainder of the ascending aorta is mildly dilated (**d**; Ao). Further quantification of LV parameters with a ventricular short-axis stack of cines demonstrated mild LV dilatation with preserved function.*

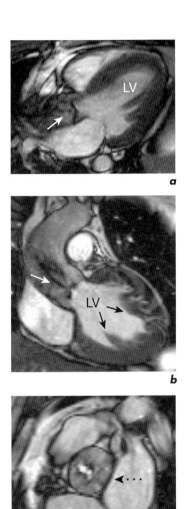

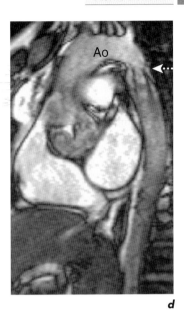

Figure 4.2 *SSFP cine CMR views from a 34-year-old man with severe AS.*
*The LVOT views (**a, b**) show marked signal loss across the AV (solid white arrows) and LVH (solid black arrows). The AV is bileaflet (**c**; dashed black arrow) and there is an associated coarctation of the aorta (**d**; dashed white arrow).*

the assessment of patients prior to valve replacement surgery, which often includes CABG and aortic root replacement. CMR also provides an excellent modality for serial surveillance of parameters such as LV function, volumes and mass in patients under follow-up and post operatively. This is done using the pre-contrast part of the protocol outlined in Chapter 1. Cines can demonstrate thickening and bulging of the aortic cusps and turbulent flow in the aorta. Imaging in an oblique sagittal plane parallel to the valve may demonstrate restricted opening and closure of the valve, and is frequently satisfactory for direct planimetry of the valve orifice and evaluation of bicuspid valve morphology. Direct planimetry can be performed using cine imaging or velocity mapping sequences (Figure 4.3).

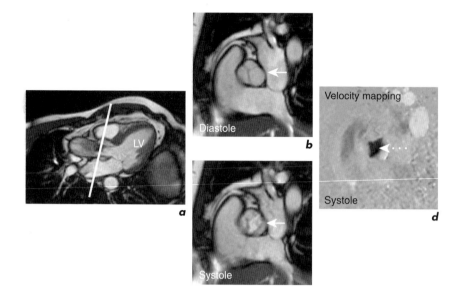

Figure 4.3 *The SSFP cine CMR LVOT view* **(a)** *allows positioning of an oblique sagittal plane just beyond the AV (white line) which then corresponds to the cine views obtained in diastole* **(b)** *and systole* **(c)** *showing bicuspid valve morphology with a fused commissure (solid white arrows). Velocity mapping in this plane* **(d)** *and these latter two images allow direct valve planimetry. However, velocity mapping is mainly used to determine the peak AV velocity. To do this, a measurement cursor is placed at several points within the valve orifice during systole (dashed white arrow) and the peak value recorded in Venc optimized images.*

Velocity mapping is primarily used, however, to calculate the pressure gradient across the AV using the modified Bernoulli equation;

$$\Delta P = 4\,(V_{max})^2$$

where ΔP (mmHg) is the pressure drop across the stenosis, and V_{max} is the peak velocity (m/s) determined by velocity mapping 1 to 1.5 cm above and parallel to the valve plane (Figure 4.3d). The typical Venc setting for the LVOT is 2 m/s, and 2.5 to 4 m/s for the aorta. An initial Venc of 2.5 m/s is often used and adjusted upwards if there is velocity aliasing (Figure 1.3). The velocity of blood flow through the AV is greater than that through the MV.

Velocity mapping, SSFP cines and FSE imaging are combined to determine the level of obstruction in AS. It is important to use information from all these sequences since a thin subaortic shelf is not reliably excluded even with high-resolution FSE CMR techniques. The initial planes and sequence required are the LVOT cines with subsequent imaging targeted by the pattern of turbulence demonstrated on these views.

Severity of AS is graded as: mild > 1.5 cm^2, moderate 1.0–1.5 cm^2, severe < 1.0 cm^2, and critical < 0.8 cm^2. In severe AS, the peak transvalvular gradient is usually > 50 mmHg.

Specific CMR reporting features for AS include:

1. Overall impression of severity (based upon peak velocity, AV area and LV function);
2. Level of stenosis; and
3. Presence or absence of associated features, such as coarctation of the aorta or aortic regurgitation (AR).

■ Aortic regurgitation

AR can be caused by valve leaflet abnormalities, dilatation of the aorta or distortion of the aortic root. Valves that are stenotic generally also have some regurgitation. Leaflet abnormalities include degeneration of a normal valve, bicuspid AV, infective endocarditis, rheumatic disease, sequelae of balloon dilatation or valvotomy for congenital AS, and thickening of the aortic cusps from the jet of subvalvular obstruction. The ascending aorta may dilate secondary to hypertension, aortitis (Reiter syndrome, ankylosing spondylitis, giant cell arteritis, relapsing polychondritis) or annuloaortic ectasia (Marfan syndrome, osteogenesis imperfecta, Ehlers–Danlos syndrome and pseudoxanthoma elasticum). Additionally, there is an aortopathy associated with bicuspid AV which causes dilatation of the ascending aorta. Distortion of the aortic root is seen with dissection, trauma and sinus of Valsalva aneurysm.

AR results in volume overload of the LV causing increased end-diastolic pressure. This is counteracted by compensatory ventricular dilatation and an increase in LV compliance which accommodates the regurgitant volume and preserves cardiac output. Patients may remain asymptomatic in this compensated phase for many years until diastolic filling pressures continue to rise and LV dysfunction or myocardial ischaemia ensue. Early detection of decompensation is critical to the timing of definitive surgical repair. Factors which influence surgical timing include severity of AR, New York Heart Association functional class, LVEF, LVESV and LVEDV, and degree of dilatation of the aortic root. In particular, LVEF and LVESV are powerful predictors of outcome in AR, and the reproducibility of these measurements as well as the reproducibility of regurgitant volume with velocity mapping CMR is excellent.

Cines in the LVOT plane demonstrate the flow void due to the regurgitant jet which can be qualitatively assessed by the size of the jet, after taking into account the effects of echo time (Figure 4.4a). Velocity mapping is performed in a plane perpendicular to the AV positioned just above the valve but below the coronary ostia (Figures 4.4b–c). This plane optimally demonstrates forward and regurgitant flow and can further characterize the morphology of the valve. The regurgitant fraction is then calculated by graphing the flow volume curve using dedicated software (Figures 4.4d–e). The area under the curve below zero in diastole represents the regurgitant volume and the regurgitant fraction is calculated by dividing this into the forward SV in systole (Figure 4.5). An alternative method is to calculate

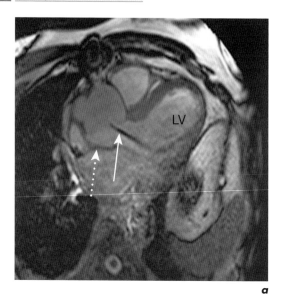

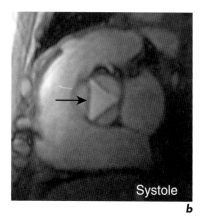

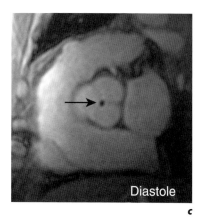

a

b

c

Figure 4.4 *SSFP cine CMR LVOT view* **(a)** *showing a central jet of AR (solid white arrow) and dilated proximal aortic root (dashed white arrow). SSFP cines in the subsequent oblique sagittal plane* **(b, c)** *show a normal trileaflet valve and confirm one central jet (black arrows) which appears black due to turbulence. This latter plane is used for the velocity mapping sequence, which in this case shows forward flow as black and regurgitant flow as white* **(d, e)**. *The region of interest is delineated throughout the cardiac cycle, in this case the AV area through systole (black circle) and diastole (white circle), and software analysis is performed to generate a curve from which the regurgitant fraction is calculated.*

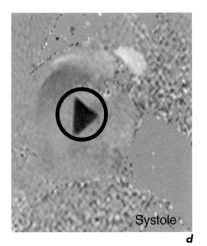

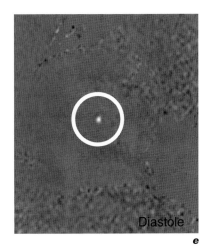

Figure 4.4 cont'd

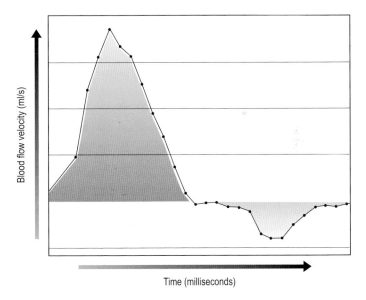

Figure 4.5 *Flow velocity time curve from the case illustrated in Figure 4.4. Using forward SV in systole (dark red) and the regurgitant volume in diastole (light red), the regurgitant fraction (regurgitant volume/SV) is automatically calculated by a dedicated software analysis tool. The value here was 20%, consistent with mild AR.*

the aortic flow and pulmonary flow at a level just above the respective valve planes. The difference in forward flow provides an estimate of the degree of AR in single-valve disease, as does the quantitative difference between RV and LVSV. The degree of ventricular dilatation also helps to qualitatively assess the severity of regurgitation. In the presence of dilatation, LGE imaging is performed to look for myocardial fibrosis, and this is especially useful in the preoperative setting.

Severity of AR by regurgitant fraction is graded as: mild < 30%, mild to moderate 30–39%, moderate to severe 40–49%, and severe > 50%.

Specific CMR reporting points for AR include:

1. Overall impression of severity (based upon jet appearance, LVEF, LVESV and LVEDV, and regurgitant fraction);
2. Dimensions of the aorta at the aortic annulus, sinuses of Valsalva, sino-tubular junction, ascending aorta (at MPA bifurcation), aortic arch, and descending thoracic aorta (at MPA bifurcation); and
3. Possible aetiology and associated features, such as dissection of the aorta and AS.

■ Mitral stenosis

Mitral stenosis (MS) is usually secondary to rheumatic heart disease. Unusual causes of MS include congenital valvular, subvalvular or supravalvular stenosis, leaflet deposits from amyloid or carcinoid, extensive mitral annular calcification and left atrial myxoma. The stenotic valve leads to a pressure gradient across the MV, causing left atrial pressures to rise. This leads to pulmonary venous hypertension and eventually to pulmonary arterial hypertension and RV failure.

CMR complements echocardiographic evaluation of MS, especially in patients with poor acoustic windows. Cines taken in the four-chamber, two-chamber and LVOT views demonstrate the thickened, hypokinetic and domed MV leaflets and a signal void arising from the MV in diastole extending into the LV (Figure 4.6). The LA is usually enlarged in moderate to severe stenosis and this is easily visualized. Additionally, the pulmonary trunk may be enlarged and tricuspid regurgitation (TR) may be present in cases with pulmonary arterial hypertension. This can be assessed in more detail by reviewing the four-chamber cine and acquiring an RVOT cine view, while a preliminary appraisal of the pulmonary arteries is readily made with the transaxial FSE acquisition. SSFP cines or velocity mapping performed in a plane parallel to the MV can be performed for direct planimetry of the stenotic valve orifice, although these can be limited by motion of the valve through the fixed imaging plane (Figure 4.7). Calculation of the valve area by direct planimetry correlates

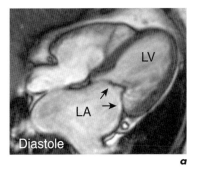 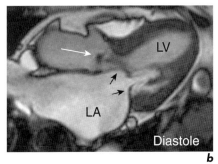

Figure 4.6 *SSFP cine images from a patient with MS secondary to rheumatic heart disease. The MV is thickened, there is turbulent inflow with limited valvular excursion (**a**; black arrows), and a dilated LA. The AV is also thickened and there is associated AR (**b**; white arrow).*

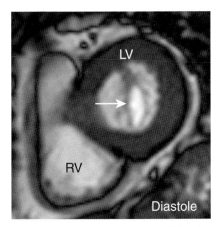

Figure 4.7 *SSFP cine image performed in a plane parallel to the MV (white arrow) from the case illustrated in Figure 4.6. Direct planimetry revealed a valve area of 1.8 cm³.*

well with echocardiographic and cardiac catheterization data, but may slightly overestimate measurements obtained by these modalities.

Velocity mapping is used to quantify the transvalvular pressure gradient using the modified Bernoulli equation, with V_{max} calculated using in-plane or preferably through-plane velocity mapping in the LV just distal to the MV. This method can underestimate the gradient. The Venc is set at a much lower value than in AS, for example 1.5 m/s.

Severity of MS is graded as: mild $\geq 1.5 \, cm^2$, moderate $1.0–1.5 \, cm^2$, and severe $< 1.0 \, cm^2$.

Specific CMR reporting points for MS include:

1. Overall impression of severity (based upon MV area, V_{max});
2. Evidence of pulmonary arterial hypertension; and
3. Associated AV involvement and mitral regurgitation (MR).

■ Mitral regurgitation

MR can be caused by abnormalities of the MV leaflets (myxomatous degeneration (Figure 4.8), rheumatic disease, endocarditis, parachute MV), chordae tendineae (myxomatous or traumatic chordal rupture, endocarditis), papillary muscle (acute infarction) or annulus (annular dilatation, periannular calcification). Chronic MR produces LA and LV dilatation due to increased SV. Pulmonary venous

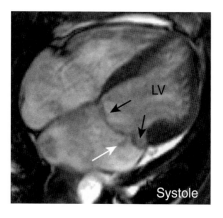

Figure 4.8 *Four-chamber SSFP cine CMR from a 40-year-old woman with familial MV prolapse (MVP). MVP is thought to be caused by myxomatous degeneration of the valve leaflets and chordae tendineae. The middle of the valve bows beyond the annulus during systole; however, the tips of the leaflets do not pass beyond this point (black arrows). Mild associated MR is noted in this case (white arrow) but is not always present.*

hypertension may be present but is usually less severe than with MS, and pulmonary arterial hypertension is also less common. Acute MR causes pulmonary venous hypertension which may be asymmetrical (right upper lobe) without atrial or ventricular enlargement.

CMR quantification of the severity of MR is useful in evaluating the signs of decompensation, monitoring response to treatment and planning MV repair or replacement. Important information required for preoperative assessment includes an EF less than 50–60% and an end-systolic diameter greater than 5.0–5.5 cm, both readily measurable with CMR. In the presence of LV dilatation or impairment, myocardial assessment with LGE is advisable.

Cines in the four-chamber, two-chamber and LVOT views demonstrate the signal void from the regurgitant jet. The jet may be central in annular dilatation or eccentric in valve leaflet, chordae tendineae or papillary muscle dysfunction. Multiple or complex jets may be present (Figure 4.9). Qualitative assessment of the severity of regurgitation can be performed by the size of the jet (accounting for the echo time) and the degree of LA dilatation. Quantification of regurgitant fraction can be performed in several ways along lines similar to that already described with AR. MR secondary to central, uncomplicated jets can be quantified by prescribing a region of interest with velocity mapping CMR using a plane placed en-face and just distal to the valve. This plane can also be used to measure effective regurgitant orifice area. A method in single regurgitant lesions is via determination of the difference in LVSV with either flow in the proximal ascending aorta or MPA, or the RVSV if no right-sided regurgitation is present.

Severity of MR by regurgitant fraction is graded as: mild < 30%, mild to moderate 30–39%, moderate to severe 40–49%, and severe > 49%.

Additional CMR reporting points for MR are:

1. Overall impression of severity (based upon jet appearance, LVEF, LVESV and LVEDV, and regurgitant fraction);
2. Evidence of pulmonary venous congestion or pulmonary arterial hypertension; and
3. Comments on aetiology and additional valvular lesions.

■ Other valve lesions

Mixed valvular disease is often present, particular in rheumatic heart disease which principally involves the MV and less commonly the AV. In late disease with pulmonary arterial hypertension, TR is also present. CMR quantification of regurgitant fractions can become complicated in this setting but is possible using velocity mapping at the individual valve planes and generating several flow velocity time curves for evaluation in comparison with LVSV and RVSV. Valve planimetry of the mitral and aortic valves can also be undertaken to yield values for an effective regurgitant orifice (Table 4.1). As with echocardiography, all available indicators of severity must be assessed collectively prior to documenting final conclusions on the clinical report.

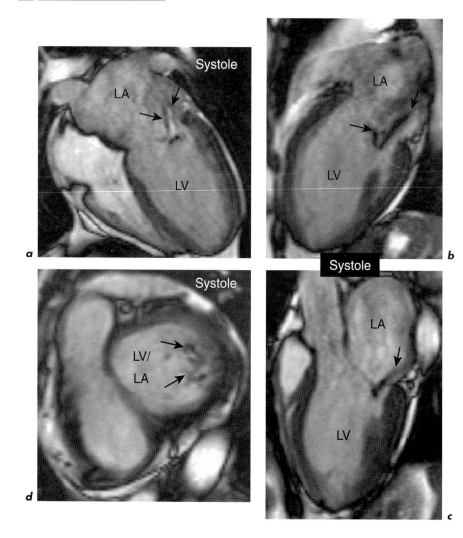

Figure 4.9 **(a)** Four-chamber, **(b)** modified two-chamber, **(c)** LVOT and **(d)** basal short-axis cines from a 42-year-old woman with multiple, eccentric jets of MR (black arrows). LVEF was 47% and regurgitant fraction calculated by comparison of LV and RV SV was 60%, indicating severe regurgitation. LGE demonstrated no enhancement.

Table 4.1 Grading of severity by effective regurgitant orifice (mm²)

Severity	MR	AR
Mild	< 20	< 10
Mild to moderate	20–29	10–19
Moderate to severe	30–39	20–29
Severe	> 40	> 30

CMR is also useful in quantifying the degree of *TR, pulmonary regurgitation* (PR) and *pulmonary stenosis* (PS). Its multiplanar capability is useful in the assessment of global RV function which may be limited using echocardiography.

Metallic prosthetic valves are safely imaged with CMR. Although assessment of paravalvular abscesses or quantification of regurgitant lesions can be performed, results may be markedly hindered by metal artefact and conclusions should therefore be interpreted within this context (Figure 4.10). FSE sequences are less affected in the presence of metal than SSFP cine or velocity mapping CMR.

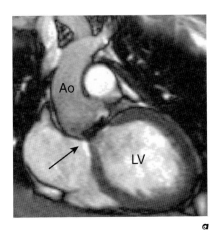
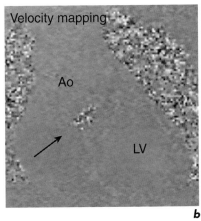

Figure 4.10 LVOT views by **(a)** SSFP cine imaging and **(b)** velocity mapping CMR in a 27-year-old woman who had undergone aortic root enlargement and AV replacement (21-mm Medtronic Hall tilting disc prosthesis) 12 years previously.
Signal void from the metal valve is clearly seen using these two sequences (black arrows), but the artefact does not preclude assessment of the valve function.

■ Indications

CMR can:

1. Image patients with poor echocardiographic windows. Although CMR assessment can be suboptimal in subjects with cardiac arrhythmias (atrial fibrillation is much less of a problem than ventricular bigeminy) and in the presence of metal valves, these should not preclude referral;
2. Arbitrate between conflicting echocardiographic and cardiac catheterization data;
3. Accurately assess the effects of valvular heart disease on cardiovascular morphology and cardiac function, and follow up these individuals; and
4. Readily interrogate right-sided valvular lesions and RV function.

CMR cannot:

1. Replace echocardiography. Echocardiography is the principal imaging modality for the initial evaluation of patients with valvular heart disease and CMR is a complementary tool;
2. Exclude small valvular vegetations in endocarditis.

Chapter 5

Cardiac masses, pericardial disease and myocarditis

Anitha Varghese and Ping Chai

■ Introduction

Detection and characterization of cardiac and pericardial masses is a Class I indication for CMR.

Imaging in constrictive pericarditis and pericardial effusion are Class II and III indications, respectively. CMR in myocarditis has an emerging role.

■ Cardiac masses

The general protocol for interrogation and subsequent reporting of masses is:

1. Anatomical evaluation—CMR can define the size, extent and anatomical relationship of masses to neighbouring structures with high resolution, across multiple planes, and with a wide field of view;
2. Cardiac functional assessment; and
3. Tissue characterization—available techniques are SE and GE sequences, application of a fat saturation prepulse, EGE and LGE, and rest perfusion CMR.

Thrombus

This is by far the commonest cardiac filling defect and both atrial and ventricular thrombi are readily visualized by SE, GE and following gadolinium (Figure 5.1). On T1W SE imaging, thrombus has intermediate signal intensity often slightly higher than myocardium and blood. T2W SE shows surrounding slow-flowing blood as having higher signal intensity than the thrombus itself, thereby enhancing differentiation from myocardium. With SSFP cine GE and velocity mapping techniques thrombus has the lowest signal intensity in distinction to blood flow, even where it is diminished, which has a high signal intensity. Injection of gadolinium contrast agent increases diagnostic accuracy and characteristically demonstrates an avascular filling defect by rest perfusion CMR and EGE. In the case of LV thrombus, subsequent LGE images usually reveal an area of infarction which has acted as the substrate for

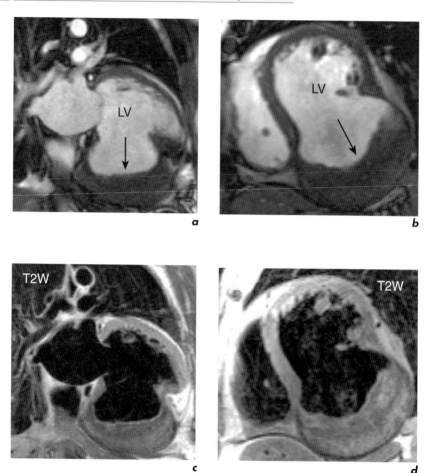

Figure 5.1 *Large inferior LV false aneurysm lined by a thick layer of laminated thrombus (black arrows) in a 70-year-old woman with a history of MI.*
(a) Two-chamber and (b) mid-ventricular short-axis SSFP GE cines show the thrombus to have much lower signal intensity than the intracavity blood flow above. Equivalent (c) two-chamber and (d) short-axis views obtained using T2W SE imaging demonstrates non-homogenous signal in the thrombus indicative of the differing stages of haemoglobin breakdown within it.

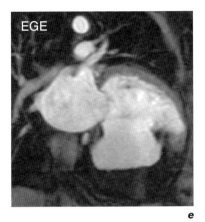
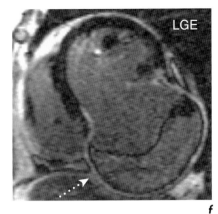

e *f*

Figure 5.1 cont'd **(e)** *Two-chamber EGE confirms an avascular filling defect surrounded inferiorly by LV transmural LGE on the ventricular short-axis view (***f***; dashed white arrow).*

thrombus formation. For atrial thrombi, a dilated LA and LA appendage can be demonstrated as with transoesophageal echocardiography (TOE).

Tumours

Secondary cardiac deposits are more frequent than primary cardiac tumours, but both are rare with a necropsy incidence of 1% and 0.05% respectively. Secondary involvement is usually clinically silent and limited to the epicardium. Presenting cardiac signs, when they occur, are those of a large pericardial effusion or incipient tamponade, arrhythmias, cardiomegaly or heart failure. Locally infiltrating malignancies include carcinoma of the lung or breast and renal cell carcinoma may embolize to the RA (Figure 5.2). Cardiac metastases are seen with malignant melanomas, leukaemias and lymphomas.

The majority of primary cardiac tumours are benign with the most frequent being atrial myxomas (45%) and cardiac lipomas (20%) (Figure 5.3). Malignant cardiac tumours make up one quarter of primary tumours and the most common are sarcomas (95%). CMR anatomical evaluation of intra- and extracardiac involvement has implications for staging, surgical treatment and surveillance (Figure 5.4). CMR differentiation between malignant and benign tumours uses a combination of general principles applied by other modalities and some more specific features. In general terms, malignancy is more likely with larger masses having a broad-based attachment, involving more than one cardiac chamber or great vessel, and with associated pericardial or extracardiac extension. More specifically, T1W and T2W images use the biochemical composition of masses to assist with diagnosis. High signal intensity on T1W images can be due to cystic lesions with a high protein content, fatty tumours (lipoma, liposarcoma), recent haemorrhage and melanoma. Low signal intensity on T1W is seen in cysts with low protein content, within vascular malformations, in calcified lesions, or if the mass contains air. Subsequent

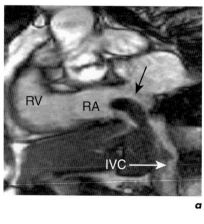

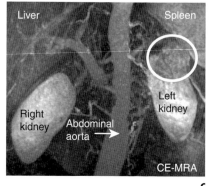

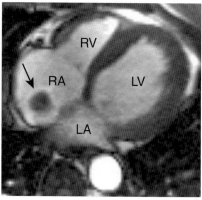

Figure 5.2 *CMR study from a 63-year-old man with left renal cell carcinoma.*
(a) SSFP GE cine image of the RA shows cardiac tumour invasion (white arrow) via the
inferior vena cava (IVC). *(b)* Transaxial SSFP GE cine confirms tumour within the RA (black
arrow). *(c)* Renal CE-MRA demonstrating a 5.5 × 4.0 × 4.5 cm³ mass in the upper half of
the left kidney (white circle).

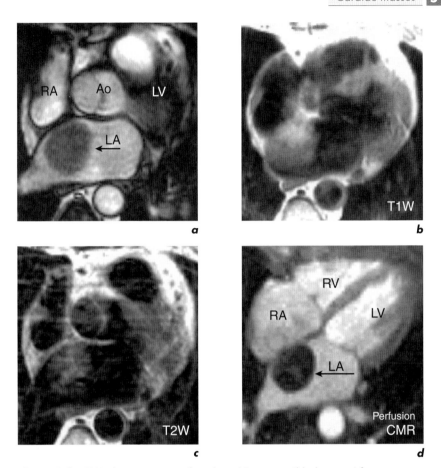

Figure 5.3 *CMR characterization of a solitary LA myxoma (black arrows) from a 65-year-old man noted to have an LA mass on TTE and TOE. **(a)** Transaxial SSFP cine GE sequence of the 4.2 × 3.8 × 4.0 cm³ ovoid mass within the LA. The base is attached to the interatrial septum and the mass has a lower signal intensity than the surrounding blood pool. **(b)** T1W SE imaging in an equivalent plane shows largely intermediate signal intensity but with a central area of increased intensity consistent with haemorrhage. **(c)** T2W imaging reveals the mass to have predominantly low signal intensity. **(d)** Four-chamber first-pass perfusion CMR demonstrates a small central core of perfusion compatible with vascularity.*
cont'd

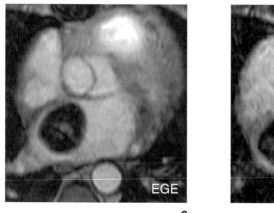
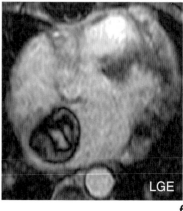

e

f

Figure 5.3 cont'd *(e)* Transaxial EGE view is largely negative but with central enhancement. *(f)* LGE in the same plane demonstrates significant enhancement, probably areas of necrosis or fibrosis.

PREOPERATIVE   POSTOPERATIVE   POST-CHEMOTHERAPY

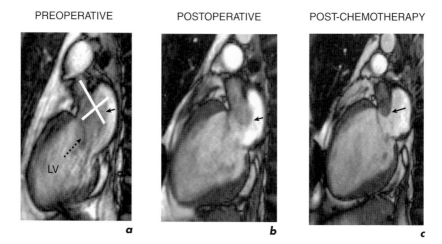

a   b   c

Figure 5.4 *Serial assessment two-chamber SSFP GE cine views from a 44-year-old man with a LA sarcoma before and after treatment (**a–c**; solid black arrows). CMR was used to accurately evaluate tumour size (**a**; white cross) and MV function (**a**; dashed black arrow) at each stage.*

T2W imaging demonstrates cysts as having high signal intensity, and the addition of a fat saturation prepulse distinguishes lipid content. Rest perfusion first-pass CMR shows contrast uptake into vascular tumours (haemangioma, angiosarcoma) and may also identify small vessels. In malignancy, EGE typically demonstrates dark areas with surrounding enhancement from necrotic tissue, while LGE can show enhancement due to expanded interstitial space such as in fibrosis (Figure 5.5). Such enhancement is absent in cystic lesions and most benign tumours, with exceptions being haemangiomas, myxomas and fibromas (Figure 5.6).

■ Pericardial disease

The pericardium is a thin double-layered sac that encompasses the heart and proximal great vessels. Its inner serosal layer adheres to the myocardium forming the visceral pericardium or epicardium, extends up over the proximal great vessels and reflects back on itself to become contiguous with the outer layer. This fibrous outer parietal layer has attachments to the diaphragm, sternum, costal cartilages and the spinal column. The two layers are separated by a space containing 15 to 35 ml of serous fluid and total pericardial thickness is 1 to 2 mm. At the base of the heart the pericardial reflection forms sinuses and recesses, with the reflection adjacent to the ascending aorta potentially confused with a proximal aortic dissection by the unwary (Figure 10.10). Since fat usually surrounds the pericardium and is also present beneath the epicardium, the pericardium is often sandwiched between two layers of fat. This makes it easier to visualize edge-on with CMR and gives the slightly higher normal value of up to 4 mm for pericardial thickness. Normal pericardium has low signal intensity by GE and SE imaging techniques (Figure 5.7). Of note, a dark line can be present at the interface between myocardium and epicardial fat on GE images due to artefact. This appearance is caused by the phenomenon of chemical shift phase cancellation and should not be interpreted as pericardium (see section 10.6, Chemical Shift Edge Artefacts).

The pericardium plays an important role in protecting and restraining the heart and has significant haemodynamic implications for atrial and ventricular filling. Because of pericardial constraint the total volume of the four cardiac chambers is limited and changes in the volume of one chamber are accompanied by opposite changes in the volume of another chamber—this effect is not physiologically important. However, when intrapericardial pressure is raised, such as in pericardial effusion, or when the pericardial cavity becomes fixed, as with constriction, the interdependence of filling between the ventricles becomes exaggerated. Intrapericardial pressure is usually similar to intrapleural pressure and with inspiration there is a small physiological increase in right heart filling and a slight decrease in left-sided filling. With increased pericardial constraint, the respiratory alterations in filling patterns become more marked.

Acute pericarditis and pericardial effusion

Acute pericarditis may be accompanied by symptoms and signs of heart failure or arrhythmias if there is concomitant myocarditis. CMR findings range from no

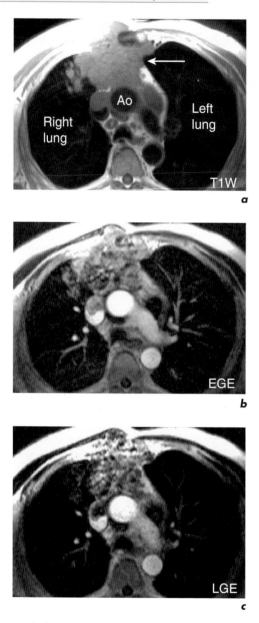

Figure 5.5 *CMR study from an 82-year-old man with TTE findings of a pericardial effusion and diastolic abnormality.*
(a) Transaxial T1W FSE demonstrates a large, irregularly shaped, highly lobulated anterior mediastinal mass (white arrow) infiltrating the sternum and chest wall anteriorly and the pericardium posteriorly. (b) EGE shows the mass to have patchy contrast uptake. (c) Patchy LGE was present. These appearances are highly suggestive of a malignancy such as lymphoma, angiosarcoma or thymic carcinoma.

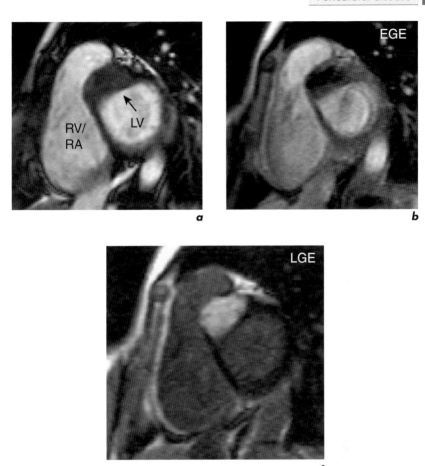

Figure 5.6 *Basal short-axis views from a 34-year-old woman referred for CMR with an echocardiographic finding of localized basal anteroseptal hypertrophy and subsequent normal cardiac biopsy.*
*Initial SSFP cine readily confirms the TTE findings (**a**; black arrow), while EGE showed no enhancement within the mass (**b**) and LGE demonstrated homogenous contrast uptake (**c**). These CMR appearances are characteristic of a fibroma.*

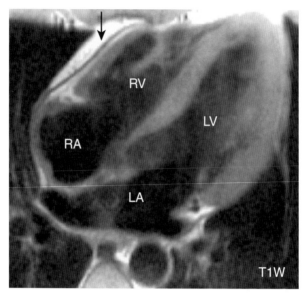

Figure 5.7 *Four-chamber T1W FSE image showing normal pericardial appearance in front of the RV (black arrow).*

abnormality to regional WMA, pericardial thickening and pericardial effusion. The heart is imaged in different planes to determine the greatest extent of thickening or effusion, especially in cases of loculation. An effusion less than 10 mm wide is considered small whereas large effusions are greater than 20 mm. Both thickened pericardium and effusions can show low signal intensity on T1W SE imaging while GE techniques reveal non-haemorrhagic effusions to have high signal intensity (Figure 5.8). The appearance of haemorrhagic effusions depends on the age of the pericardial haematoma. Acutely, there is high signal intensity on T1W SE and lower signal intensity on GE images, while more chronic haematomas exhibit heterogeneous signal intensities by SE techniques. Differentiation of transudates from exudates and chylous effusions is through T1W SE imaging. Signal intensity is low in transudates but high in chylous collections, with an intermediate appearance in exudates.

SSFP GE cine imaging demonstrates diastolic chamber collapse and abnormal septal motion in cardiac tamponade. In the latter, the heart can often have a swinging motion. Other pathological findings include dilated superior and inferior vena cavae and the presence of abnormalities within the mediastinum and lung fields which could provide clues as to aetiology.

Following gadolinium injection, inflamed pericardium shows early enhancement with a smooth contour suggestive of acute pericarditis in contrast to an irregular outline after a more insidious clinical course. Such pericardial contrast enhancement is also seen in malignant infiltration. Contrast enhancement is usually absent in pericardial fluid.

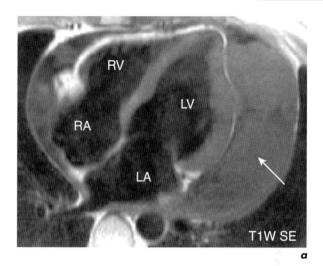

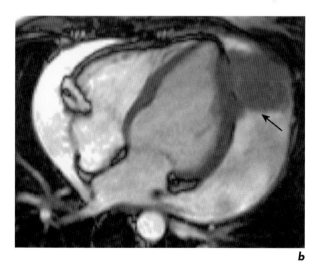

Figure 5.8 *Four-chamber views from a 42-year-old woman with a large global pericardial effusion (**a**; white arrow) secondary to metastatic leiomyosarcoma (**b**; black arrow). The effusion is seen to have intermediate signal intensity by SE imaging (**a**) and a high signal intensity using the GE technique, which clearly shows the tumour (**b**).*

With massive effusion, ECG amplitude may diminish making it difficult to trigger cardiac imaging. CMR assessment can also be limited in patients who are significantly symptomatic since they have a tachycardia and find it difficult to lie flat within the magnet for prolonged periods.

Constrictive pericarditis

Following inflammation or bleeding into the pericardial space, fibrosis and calcification of the pericardium may ensue and the pericardium becomes thickened and stiff. This progressively restricts and impairs the filling of the cardiac chambers. Diastolic pressures are elevated and equalized in all four cardiac chambers. Impaired diastolic function leads to tachycardia and volume expansion, resulting in systemic venous congestion. Systolic function is usually preserved unless there is associated myocardial disease. The heart is insulated from changes in intrathoracic pressure that occur with respiration and atrial and ventricular filling patterns vary significantly with inspiration and expiration, resulting in ventricular interdependence. During inspiration, right-sided filling is increased, the ventricular septum deviates to the left, and left-sided filling correspondingly decreases. The converse occurs at expiration.

The distinction between constrictive pericarditis and restrictive cardiomyopathy is difficult but important clinically and imaging techniques such as CMR and cardiac CT are useful in diagnosis. The diagnostic hallmark of constrictive pericarditis is pericardial thickening with or without calcification in the presence of suggestive symptoms and signs of constriction (Figure 5.9). Care should be taken when evaluating pericardial thickness since oblique views yield falsely high values and several planes must be assessed and used in measurements. The absence of pericardial thickening/calcification does not exclude the presence of constriction and a thickened

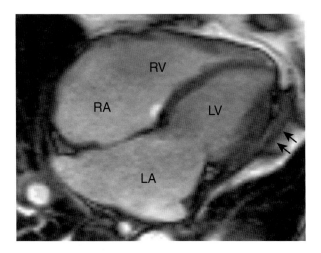

Figure 5.9 *Four-chamber SSFP GE cine view from an 81-year-old woman with a history of recurrent pericardial effusions requiring surgical drainage and features of constrictive pericarditis at recent cardiac catheterization.*
There is bi-atrial dilatation and a thickened pericardium (black arrows), which measured 9 mm in this plane. No pericardial effusion is seen and LVEF was 68% (normal).

pericardium does not always equate to constrictive pericarditis. It is therefore crucial to evaluate concomitant functional consequences and CMR is well-suited for this purpose.

A thickened pericardium as well as pericardial effusions can often be identified at the early low-resolution FSE sequence. Pericardial thickness is definitively measured on subsequent T1W FSE views and differentiated from effusion with SSFP cines acquired in these same planes. In the presence of effusion, pericardial thickness can be determined by use of gadolinium which can outline the visceral and parietal layers. Chronic fibrotic pericardium shows late enhancement, which is also seen with associated myocardial fibrosis or infarction. Areas of calcification appear as regions of attenuated signal intensity on CMR but CT is recommended for accurate assessment of this feature. Other findings include typically normal-sized or small ventricles with normal ejection fraction, dilated atria and vena cavae, pleural effusions, plethoric hepatic veins, hepatic enlargement and ascites. The ventricles may assume a tube-like configuration. The presence of epicardial fat separating the epimyocardium from the thickened visceral pericardium is also a useful finding for the surgeon when planning surgical pericardiectomy.

On high temporal resolution SSFP cines, the ventricular septum may be seen to deviate towards the LV in early diastole. Additional real-time cines are useful in demonstrating ventricular interdependence. The patient is instructed to inhale and exhale throughout these cines, which are acquired over approximately 20s and at least three respiratory cycles. With constrictive physiology, the ventricular septum flattens and deviates towards the LV on inspiration before resuming its normal position on expiration—'septal bounce'. The technique of myocardial tagging can determine myocardial tethering to the overlying thickened pericardium with persistent concordance of the tag lines between myocardium and pericardium throughout systole and diastole.

In summary, a suggested CMR imaging protocol in significant pericardial effusion/constriction is as follows:

- Multislice free breathing FSE in transaxial, coronal and sagittal planes;
- SSFP cines in the usual views, selected transaxial and sagittal planes, and additional planes through areas of abnormal pericardium or loculated effusion;
- T1W FSE imaging of the views in which abnormalities are identified;
- Gadolinium-enhanced SE and GE imaging of the views in which the pericardium is abnormal; and
- If constriction is suspected:
  — High temporal resolution SSFP cines of the four-chamber and mid-ventricular short-axis views;
  — Real-time SSFP cines of the mid-ventricular short-axis view; and
  — Myocardial tagged cine images of the views in which thickened pericardium is identified.

CMR reports include:

1. Anatomical details—such as cardiac chamber size, vena cavae dilatation, pericardial thickness, presence and characterization of effusions (especially in terms of size, loculation and suggested sites for safe pericardiocentesis if required) and pleural effusions;
2. Cardiac functional comments—such as evidence of cardiomyopathy and tamponade physiology; and
3. Clues to aetiology—such as contrast enhancement patterns within the pericardium and myocardium.

Pericardial cyst and diverticula

Pericardial cysts are uncommon remnants of defective pericardial embryologic development. They are benign and occur as round, sharply demarcated, fluid-filled bodies, found most commonly in the right cardiophrenic angle but also in the hilar and mediastinal regions. They do not communicate with the pericardial space. Using T2W SE images they typically exhibit high signal intensity, while on T1W SE images they show intermediate or low signal intensities (Figure 5.10). There is no enhancement with gadolinium contrast.

Pericardial diverticula are rare outpouchings of the pericardial sac and therefore are in communication with the pericardial space.

Congenital absence of the pericardium

Absence of the pericardium is rare and often asymptomatic. The defect is usually left-sided and partial but can be right-sided, diaphragmatic or complete. Associated congenital cardiac anomalies include atrial septal defects (ASDs), patent ductus arteriosus (PDA) and tetralogy of Fallot (TOF). The heart shifts to the left and posteriorly, and with partial left-sided absence the left atrial appendage may be dilated. Herniation of the left atrial appendage through a partial defect may lead to strangulation and sudden death. CMR can reveal the defect, associated cardiac anomalies and displacement, and herniation (Figure 5.11).

■ Myocarditis

Myocarditis can be caused by a wide variety of infectious agents and detected with the technique of LGE. Patterns of enhancement do not correspond to infarction in a coronary artery territory and are characteristically subepicardial and frequently located in the lateral free wall (Figure 5.12). These appearances in conjunction with the appropriate clinical setting can obviate the necessity for cardiac catheterization and subsequent endomyocardial biopsy in selected patients. Follow-up of individuals with significant enhancement abnormalities, with either echocardiography or CMR, is also advisable to determine long-term ventricular function.

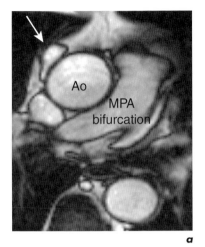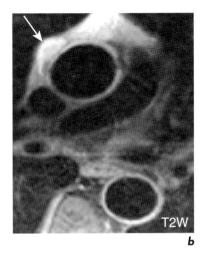

Figure 5.10 *An incidental finding of a small 2.6 × 1.8 × 5 cm³ pericardial cyst (white arrows) discovered in a 71-year-old man referred for coronary MRA showing characteristic high signal intensity by **(a)** SSFP cine and **(b)** T2W SE imaging in a transaxial plane at the level of the pulmonary bifurcation.*

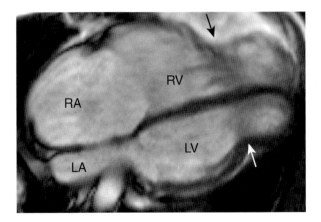

Figure 5.11 *Four-chamber SSFP GE cine image from a 46-year-old patient demonstrating herniation of both ventricles through a partially absent pericardium at the level arrowed.*
There is associated RA and RV dilatation on this image secondary to severe TR which is not shown.

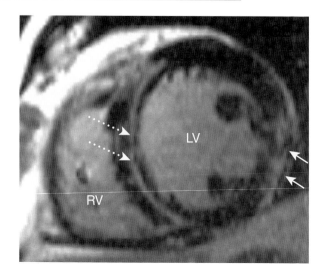

Figure 5.12 *LGE in a mid-ventricular short-axis plane from a 61-year-old man with long-standing anterolateral ST segment changes but no significant CAD at X-ray coronary angiography. Enhancement is seen within the mid-wall of the interventricular septum (dashed white arrows) and subepicardial aspect of the lateral wall (solid white arrows). This pattern in association with a dilated LV and impaired LVEF (28%) was suggestive of a myocarditis-induced cardiomyopathy.*

■ Indications

CMR can:

1. Detect and characterize cardiac masses including atrial and ventricular thrombi;
2. Be used to stage malignant cardiac tumours;
3. Safely be used in oncology surveillance;
4. Detect and characterize pericardial effusions;
5. Detect pericardial constriction;
6. Demonstrate abnormal haemodynamics of increased intrapericardial pressures, such as ventricular interdependence;
7. Detect and characterize pericardial masses;
8. Diagnose congenital abnormalities of the pericardium and associated cardiac defects; and
9. Accurately diagnose myocarditis.

CMR cannot:

1. Readily image patients who have severe dyspnoea and tachycardia due to scan positioning and duration, and imaging artefacts from respiratory and cardiac motion; and
2. Exclude pericardial calcification.

Chapter 6

Diseases of the aorta

Beatriz Bouzas

■ Introduction

The aorta can be evaluated by a variety of techniques (Figure 6.1). X-ray contrast angiography was the gold standard method for many years but it is invasive and uses ionizing radiation and nephrotoxic contrast agents. Noninvasive options are TOE, CT and CMR (Figure 6.2). TOE is portable but relatively invasive and offers

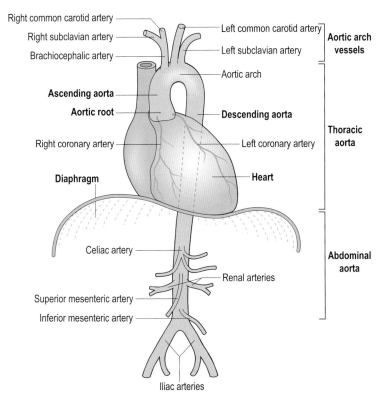

Figure 6.1 *Diagrammatic representation of the normal aorta.*

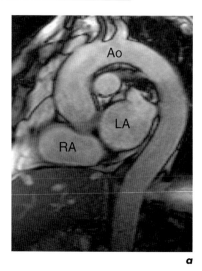
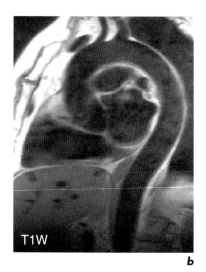

Figure 6.2 *Normal CMR study of the aorta from a 60-year-old man referred for further investigation of hypertension with a family history of an ascending aortic aneurysm and marfanoid features.*

*These images show the oblique sagittal plane (known as the 'hockey-stick' or 'candy cane' view) from which several measurements can often be made using the **(a)** GE or **(b)** SE sequence. This aortic long-axis view is a plane obtained from the initial transaxial FSE images by placement of three markers—at the ascending aorta, at the aortic arch and at the descending thoracic aorta. Quoted aortic dimensions are usually intraluminal, at end-diastole, and should state clearly the sequence used in order to facilitate serial evaluation.*

incomplete coverage of the aorta with restricted visualization at the aortic arch. CT is fast and widely available but uses ionizing radiation and nephrotoxic contrast agents. CMR avoids these limitations and offers multiplanar imaging of the aorta with a wide field of view and concurrent cardiac functional assessment. However, it is less available and evaluation of critically ill patients can be hampered by MRI-incompatible life support and monitoring equipment.

CMR reports of scans pertaining to the aorta follow the general pattern of:

(a) Anatomical details of the heart and aorta;
(b) Concurrent cardiac functional assessment, for example quantification of AR and degree of LVH; and
(c) Likely aetiology of aortic pathology with suggestions for follow-up.

■ Thoracic aortic aneurysm

An aortic aneurysm is a focal dilatation of the aorta. According to the shape the aneurysm is described as fusiform, with symmetrical dilatation of the circumference of the aorta, or saccular where only a part of the aortic wall is dilated. Aortic aneurysms can also be classified into true and false aneurysms. A true aneurysm consists of dilatation of all the layers of the aortic wall and characteristically has a wide neck. By contrast, in a false aneurysm perforation of the intima and media is contained by the surrounding adventitia and peri-aortic tissue, and the neck is usually narrow.

Aortic aneurysms are usually the consequence of atherosclerotic disease and most commonly occur at the descending aorta (Figure 6.3). Other causes are trauma, connective tissue disorders such as Marfan and Ehlers–Danlos syndromes, congenital abnormalities, and infections such as syphilis. Post-stenotic aneurysms are found distal to AV stenosis and aortic coarctation or recoarctation.

CMR can readily detect aortic aneurysms and scan protocols evaluate the following:

- Aneurysm location, shape, 3D size, and extension;
- Involvement of the AV and aortic root (including coronary arteries);
- Proximity to branch vessels (such as the left subclavian, renal and iliac arteries);
- Presence of intraluminal flow and thrombus;
- Associated aortic dissection; and
- Pericardial effusions (Figure 6.4).

SE images acquired in the transverse and long-axis planes are useful for measuring the diameter of the aorta at different levels and relationship of the aneurysm to major vessels. Coronal and oblique sagittal views clearly depict the aortic root and tortuous segments. Slow or turbulent blood flow can produce images which mimic mural thrombus on SE imaging. SSFP cines and velocity flow mapping help to differentiate slow flow from intraluminal thrombus. Where intraluminal thrombus

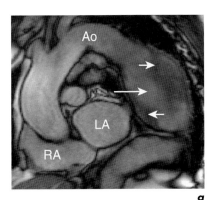
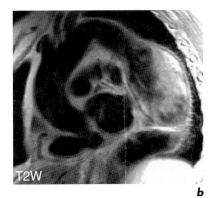

a   *b*

Figure 6.3 *Hockey-stick (**a**) SSFP cine and (**b**) T2W SE views from a 74-year-old man with a 6.2 cm fusiform descending thoracic aortic aneurysm (large white arrow) containing a large amount of mural thrombus (small white arrows).*

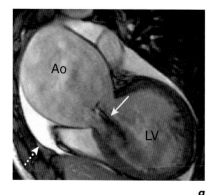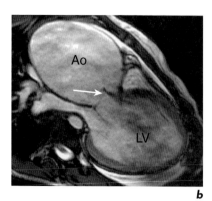

a b

Figure 6.4 *LVOT SSFP GE cines from a 20-year-old man with Marfan syndrome showing an 11.5 cm ascending aortic aneurysm (Ao) associated with severe AR (solid white arrows), dilated LV, and a small global pericardial effusion (dashed white arrows). There was no evidence of dissection.*

is present, its thickness and extent should be determined. CMR allows characterization of intraluminal thrombus based on signal changes caused by the paramagnetic properties of deoxyhaemoglobin and methaemoglobin. Methaemoglobin forms from red blood cell lysis and shortens T1 but increases T2, causing hyperintensity on both T1W and T2W SE sequences. Thrombus with homogeneous low signal intensity on both T1W and T2W images corresponds to macroscopic organized thrombus. Some organized thrombi may have an internal rim of hyperintensity which represents recent clot apposition on the luminal surface of the thrombus. Thrombi with homogeneous high signal intensity on T1W and T2W imaging represent unorganized thrombi, composed mainly of fresh clot. Some thrombi may appear partially organized, with areas of high and low signal intensity (Figure 6.5). Inflammatory aortic aneurysms may show an area of peri-aortic inflammation that enhances following gadolinium contrast. This can be better visualized using a T1W CMR sequence with an added fat saturation prepulse. MRA is useful for assessing aortic flow and involvement and patency of aortic branch vessels. Images are acquired in the aortic long-axis plane and can then be reformatted into the transaxial plane. Post-processing techniques, such as maximum intensity projections (MIPs) and shaded surface displays, are used for representation (Figure 6.6). CMR is useful for follow-up evaluation of aneurysm size and serial measurements must be made at the same level.

Percutaneous stent-graft placement has emerged in the recent years as an effective way of treating aortic aneurysms and dissection. CMR is useful in planning these interventions allowing customization of stent design according to aortic anatomy, and detection of post-stent leaks. Accurate quantification of aortic calcification prior to stenting requires CT rather than CMR.

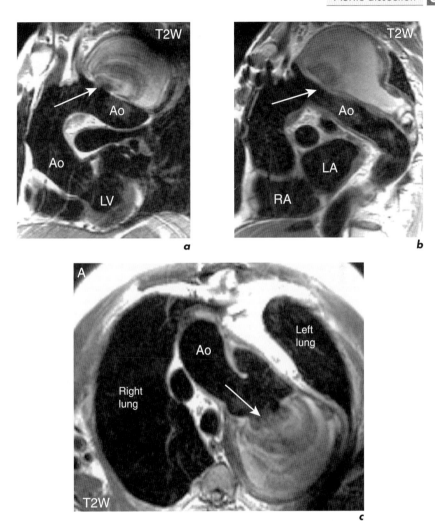

Figure 6.5 *Modified **(a)** coronal, **(b)** sagittal and **(c)** transaxial T2W SE planes from a 70-year-old woman demonstrate a 10 × 10 × 6 cm³ aortic arch pseudoaneurysm on the outer curvature of the distal aortic arch containing partially organized mural thrombus (white arrows).*

■ Aortic dissection

Aortic dissection consists of an intimal flap separating the true and false lumen, and intimal tears are sites of communication between the true and false lumen. A dissection can spread antegradely or retrogradely and may involve the whole length of the aorta. It can lead to occlusion or obstruction of branch vessels, aortic regurgitation and pericardial effusion. Aetiology includes hypertension (the most common), atherosclerosis, congenital lesions, iatrogenic causes and trauma.

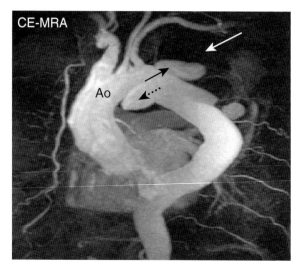

Figure 6.6 *MIP reconstruction of the CE-MRA data obtained from the case illustrated in Figure 6.5.*
Of note, the large outer aortic arch pseudoaneurysm (white arrow) is clearly seen to be in communication with the aortic lumen via a 2.5 cm entry site (solid black arrow). Additionally, a second, smaller pseudoaneurysm (3.5 × 2.3 × 6.0 cm³) is demonstrated on the inner aortic arch (dashed black arrow).

Aortic dissections are classified by the De Bakey or Stanford classification system. The De Bakey classification is based on the location of the intimal tear and the extent of the dissection:

Type I: Intimal tear originates in the ascending aorta and extends past the origin of the left subclavian artery.

Type II: Intimal tear originates in the ascending aorta and the dissection is limited to the ascending aorta.

Type III: Intimal tear originates beyond the origin of the left subclavian artery and extends distally.

The Stanford classification is based on prognosis and has implications for management.

Type A: Dissection involves the ascending thoracic aorta (Figure 6.7).

Type B: Dissection does not involve the ascending thoracic aorta (Figure 6.8).

Type A dissection carries a higher complication rate and mortality and is a surgical emergency, while type B dissections have a better prognosis and are usually managed medically.

CMR is the gold standard imaging technique for detecting and characterizing aortic dissections with their associated complications in the haemodynamically stable patient. Scan protocols evaluate the following after diagnosis:

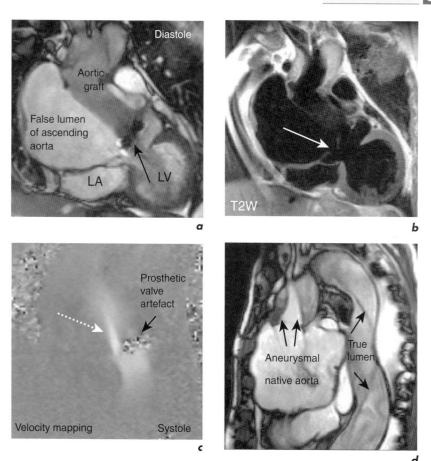

Figure 6.7 CMR study from a 57-year-old man who had undergone aortic root and valve repair the previous year, followed by AV replacement with a metal prosthetic valve. At follow-up a dilated ascending aortic aneurysm and AR were noted. **(a)** LVOT SSFP cine confirms an aneurysmal ascending aorta with false lumen between native aorta and aortic graft. Dehiscence of the posterior suture line of the prosthetic AV resulted in a rocking motion of the valve and severe paravalvular regurgitation (long black arrow).
(b) Comparative T2W SE image highlighting the suture line dehiscence (solid white arrow).
(c) Velocity mapping CMR in the same plane showing blood flowing freely between the LV and false lumen (dashed white arrow). **(d)** Oblique sagittal SSFP GE aortic cine showing dissection flaps in the proximal aortic arch and the descending thoracic aorta (short black arrows).

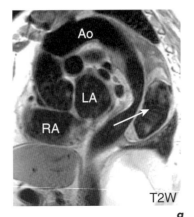

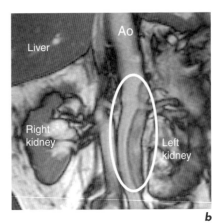

a

b

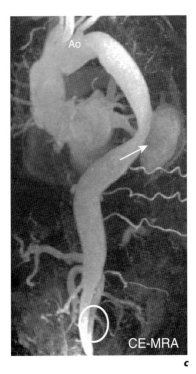

c

Figure 6.8 *Residual type B aortic dissection from a 67-year-old man who had undergone repair of a type A dissection one year previously.*
(a) Oblique sagittal T2W SE shows the false lumen of the thoracic dissection (white arrow). This extends from 4 cm beyond the left subclavian artery to 2 cm above the diaphragm and is largely thrombosed with evidence of a fresh inner layer of thrombus. (b) Oblique coronal SSFP cine demonstrates the abdominal dissection (white ellipse). (c) MIP reconstruction of the CE-MRA data showing the two separate dissections (white arrow and white ellipse). Both renal arteries receive flow from the true lumen.

- Location of proximal intimal flap and involvement of the ascending aorta, AV, and coronary arteries;
- Extension of dissection and sites of entry and re-entry (intimal tear);
- Presence of thrombus within the false lumen;
- Involvement of branch vessels with a comment on which lumen supplies them; and
- Associated pericardial and pleural effusions.

SE imaging delineates the intimal flap as a linear structure separating the true and false lumens. Slow flow (usually within the false lumen) or thrombus is differentiated by SSFP cines in the same plane. Cines are useful in detecting AR, and both sequences help in the diagnosis of pericardial effusions. Velocity mapping CMR also distinguishes diminished flow from intraluminal thrombus and highlights flow directionality in the false lumen (antegrade/retrograde). AR, where present, is quantified by velocity mapping in the appropriate plane. CE–MRA shows the flap and branch vessel involvement.

■ Intramural haematomas and penetrating aortic ulcers

An intramural haematoma has a similar clinical presentation and prognosis to that of aortic dissection and is also associated with arterial hypertension. It is thought to be caused by spontaneous rupture of the aortic vasa vasorum with subsequent propagation of subintimal haemorrhage, and there is a high rate of progression to aortic dissection and risk of aortic wall rupture. By contrast to dissections, there is more frequent involvement of the descending aorta and less frequent AR, MI and pulse deficits since they are more localized. The location of intramural haematomas carries prognostic and management implications with those in the ascending aorta having a higher frequency of complications and requiring surgical treatment.

Intramural haematomas are characterized by the presence of intramural blood and/or increased arterial wall thickness which can be asymmetrical or circumferential (Figure 6.9). T1W and T2W SE imaging allows some determination of the age of the haemorrhage. Acutely (first 5–7 days) intramural haematoma appears as increased wall thickness of intermediate signal intensity which is isodense with the aortic wall. Subacutely (more than 8 days) there is high signal intensity similar to fat due to the presence of methaemoglobin. Transaxial planes should be acquired in preference to longitudinal views due to improved differentiation from mediastinal fat. Addition of a fat saturation prepulse sequence further improves distinction between haematoma and fat. MRA will usually not detect intramural haematomas since there is no luminal component.

Penetrating aortic ulcers consist of an intimal erosion penetrating the aortic wall from within the aortic lumen. There is an association with intramural haematoma and a risk of progression to aortic dissection or perforation. MRA reveals a focal area of contrast extravasation communicating with the aortic lumen. Penetrating ulcers are found predominantly in the descending thoracic and abdominal aorta, with the most frequent risk factor being aortic atherosclerosis.

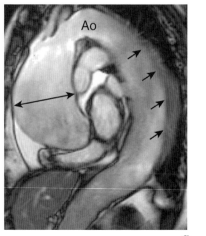
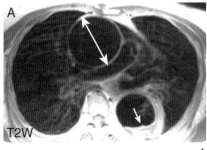

Figure 6.9 *(a) Oblique sagittal SSFP cine view of the aorta and (b) transaxial T2W SE image from a 79-year-old man with chronic hypertension, aneurysm of the ascending aorta (two-headed arrows) and extensive intramural haematoma of the distal aortic arch and descending thoracic aorta (single-headed arrows).*

■ Aortitis

Takayasu arteritis is a granulomatous vasculitis of unknown aetiology that commonly affects the thoracic and abdominal aorta. Inflammation leads to thickening of the aortic wall and the origin of the main branches, mainly in the aortic arch, with sequelae including aortic branch thrombosis, stenosis or occlusion. The pulmonary arteries can also be affected. SE imaging demonstrates diffuse wall thickening and MRA provides good visualization of aneurysm formation and branch vessel stenosis and/or occlusion.

■ Marfan syndrome

Marfan syndrome is an inherited connective tissue disorder with significant cardiovascular, skeletal and ocular system complications. CMR evaluates:

- Mitral and tricuspid valve (TV) prolapse;
- Aortic root dilatation;
- Ascending and descending thoracic aortic aneurysm formation; and
- Presence of aortic dissection.

Aortic dissection and rupture account for most deaths in this condition and affected individuals undergo regular CMR surveillance of the aorta to help plan elective aortic root replacement. Aortic root dimension and the rate of increase are the best predictors of those at greatest risk of aortic dissection, and prophylactic root replacement is recommended before diameters reach 55–60 mm. In patients with family history of aortic dissection, replacement is performed when the aortic root measures 50 mm. Progressive thoracoabdominal vasculopathy postoperatively necessitates continued follow-up after repair of the ascending aorta. Patients with an aortic dissection or peripheral artery aneurysms require more frequent CMR assessment.

■ Coarctation of the aorta

Coarctation of the aorta occurs in approximately 1 in 10000 people and is usually diagnosed in children or adults under 40 years old. It commonly consists of a stenosis of the aorta just distal to the origin of the left subclavian artery. The area of coarctation can be a localized narrowing or a long hypoplastic segment involving the aortic arch and descending thoracic aorta. Haemodynamically significant lesions are associated with the development of collaterals from the intercostal, internal mammary and anterior spinal arteries which then can supply blood to the descending aorta (Figure 6.10). Bicuspid AV is frequently seen with aortic coarctation and this cohort can progress to AS or AR. Dilatation of the ascending aorta may precede aortic aneurysm formation and type A aortic dissection in these patients.

CMR is the imaging modality of choice in adult aortic coarctation. The study evaluates:

- Site, extent and degree of aortic coarctation;
- Flow across the stenosis and assessment of severity;
- Collateral blood flow;
- Associated cardiovascular complications such as bicuspid AV and dilated ascending aorta; and
- Results of childhood and adult interventions.

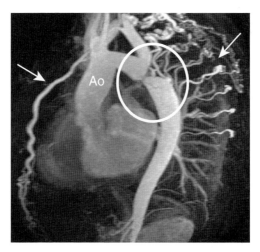

Figure 6.10 *MIP reconstruction of CE-MRA data in the oblique sagittal view from a 25-year-old woman showing discrete coarctation of the aorta just distal to the left subclavian artery pre-catheter intervention (white circle). Associated internal mammary and intercostal artery collaterals are arrowed.*

The oblique sagittal plane is imaged using SE and SSFP cines for assessment of anatomy, but several other planes may be required with increased tortuosity. Blood flow across the stenosis is recognized with cines and these are then used to position the planes required for velocity mapping CMR. Flow velocity mapping techniques across the coarctation measure blood flow velocity and a pressure gradient is then estimated with the modified Bernoulli formula. Resting peak velocity of greater than 3 m/s is significant, particularly in the presence of diastolic prolongation of forward flow—a diastolic tail. Flow velocities may normalize in significant coarctation with extensive collateralization. The percentage of collateral blood flow is calculated from measurements of flow just proximal to the coarctation site and within the descending thoracic aorta at the level of the diaphragm. Collateral blood flow is significantly increased in severe coarctation. MRA readily demonstrates tortuosity, involvement of aortic arch vessels and presence of collaterals.

Long-term outcomes following elective intervention in coarctation are optimal when performed at 2–5 years of age. Late complications include hypertension, re-stenosis, residual stenosis and aneurysm formation. CMR is performed at baseline post-intervention and then at intervals thereafter, depending on clinical and imaging findings (Figures 6.11 and 6.12). Haemoptysis in a patient with coarctation may indicate leakage of blood through a false aneurysm. Serial contiguous SE sequences should be used in this situation to identify bright para-aortic haematoma.

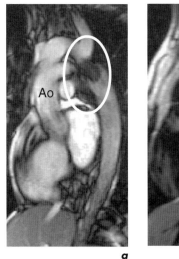 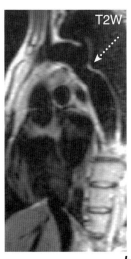 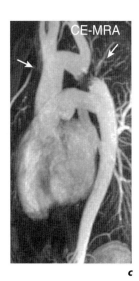

a *b* *c*

Figure 6.11 *One-year post-catheter intervention CMR study of the patient in Figure 6.10. Oblique sagittal views show mild residual in-stent stenosis.*
(a) SSFP cine reveals metallic stent artefact at the site of previous coarctation (white ellipse). Subsequent flow velocity mapping CMR performed distal to the stent demonstrated increased systolic velocity without a diastolic tail. (b) T2W SE images improve the stent artefact and allow measurement of the reduced minimum in-stent diameter (dashed white arrow). (c) MIP reconstruction of CE-MRA data shows reduced collateralization (white arrows).

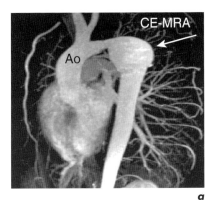 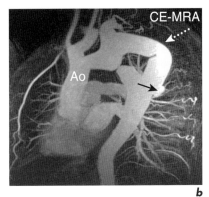

Figure 6.12 *Two examples of postoperative aneurysm formation shown using MIPs displayed in the oblique sagittal plane.*
(a) CE-MRA from a 19-year-old man who had undergone repair of aortic coarctation with a subclavian flap and Impra patch aged 3. There is a fusiform aneurysm (solid white arrow) distal to mild recoarctation at the mid-aortic arch. (b) CE-MRA from a 51-year-old man who had undergone aortic coarctation repair with a Gelseal graft placed between the dilated left subclavian artery and descending thoracic aorta (dashed white arrow). There is a small, contained false aneurysm at the distal suture line of the graft (black arrow).

■ Rare congenital anomalies of the aorta

A *right-sided aortic arch* consists of a single aortic arch located to the right of the trachea. This congenital anomaly is associated with TOF and truncus arteriosus. A *double aortic arch* refers to persistence of both the right and left aortic arch leading to the formation of a vascular ring around the trachea and oesophagus. This ring may compress these structures, causing dyspnoea and dysphagia. An *aberrant origin of the right subclavian artery* from the descending aorta may also cause airways compromise due to direct compression as it crosses obliquely towards the right shoulder behind the trachea.

CMR with SE and cines permits rapid evaluation of the anatomy of aortic arch anomalies and their relationship to surrounding structures. Associated congenital cardiovascular anomalies must also be characterized during the study. MRA allows easy visualization of the anomaly from different orientations and is an excellent way of communicating these unusual findings to colleagues.

■ Indications

CMR can:

1. Diagnose thoracic aortic aneurysms, aortic dissection, aortic intramural haematoma and penetrating ulcers of the aorta, coarctation (and pseudocoarctation) of the aorta, and rare congenital anomalies of the aorta;

2. Readily follow-up these cases and patients with Marfan syndrome pre- and post-intervention. Metallic artefacts will affect images but do not preclude useful CMR evaluation;
3. Assist planning for intervention;
4. Differentiate aortic dissection from intramural haematomas and penetrating aortic ulcers; and
5. Perform concurrent cardiac anatomical and functional evaluation.

CMR cannot:

1. Reliably detect calcification within the aortic wall; and
2. Be recommended for the assessment of acute aortic pathology in haemodynamically unstable patients.

Chapter 7

Adult congenital heart disease

Richard Steeds

■ Introduction

Congenital heart disease has an incidence of approximately 1% (Figure 7.1). Advances in medical and surgical management have resulted in a growing population of young adults who require continued care due to the predominantly palliative rather than curative nature of their interventions. CMR provides safe serial assessment of patients with adult congenital heart disease (ACHD).

> CMR can often differentiate patients in whom cardiac catheterization can be deferred and delineate the management required. This reduces the number of diagnostic invasive procedures and helps optimize interventions.

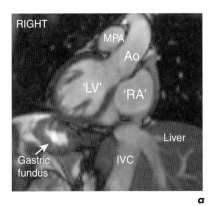
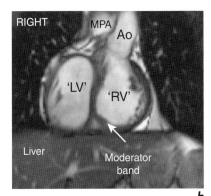

a   b

Figure 7.1 *Two cases of dextrocardia.*
(a) 'LVOT' SSFP cine view from a 42-year-old woman showing situs inversus with dextrocardia. Situs inversus occurs more commonly with dextrocardia than with levocardia. A 3–5% incidence of congenital heart disease is observed in situs inversus with dextrocardia, usually with transposition of the great vessels, while situs inversus with levocardia is almost always associated with congenital heart disease. (b) Coronal SSFP GE cine view from a 40-year-old man with situs solitus and dextrocardia. There is associated congenitally corrected transposition of the great arteries (ccTGA).

CMR images and measurements complement those obtained using echocardiography, especially in postoperative patients. Accurate anatomical and functional information of complex cardiac pathology can be obtained in any plane. These factors make pre- and post-intervention CMR evaluation in ACHD invaluable.

■ CMR protocol

Standard CMR protocols in ACHD are centred on evaluation of cardiac morphology and cardiac function with interrogation of stenoses, regurgitant jets, shunt patency and chamber performance. MRA and myocardial tissue characterization are of increasing importance. Scan reports comment on:

1. Cardiac chamber size;
2. Quantitative values for biventricular function and mass; and
3. Detailed characterization of abnormalities of flow.

Other reporting requirements are highlighted following discussion of specific conditions.

Cardiac morphology and function

Breath-hold SE imaging with multislice transaxial FSE followed by multislice SSFP in all three orthogonal planes (transaxial, coronal and sagittal) is useful for optimal planning of subsequent planes. Adequate anatomical coverage is preserved despite the temporal limitation imposed by breath-holding using staggered acquisition of contiguous slices and allowing breathing in-between, or additional software which speeds up the scan further at the expense of resolution. In the presence of significant metallic artefact FSE acquisitions are degraded to a lesser degree than GE sequences.

Subsequent cines are acquired in planes determined by the underlying diagnosis and provide higher resolution anatomical and functional information on parameters including biventricular size, function and mass. Assessment of the RV and pulmonary vasculature is of particular importance in ACHD along with extensive flow velocity mapping for measurement of peak velocities, regurgitant fractions and shunt performance (Figure 7.2). The Venc is set to account for low velocities in venous systems and higher velocities within shunts. Information from both the cines and velocity mapping is crucial for interpretation of the patterns of blood flow. Cine images also direct optimal positioning of velocity mapping sequences.

Contrast use

MRA with gadolinium is useful for the assessment of pulmonary branch artery, aortic and major arterial anatomy. The LGE technique is being increasingly used to identify ischaemic or post-surgical scarring of ventricular myocardium.

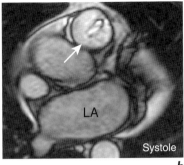

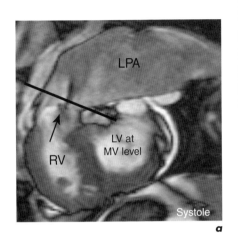

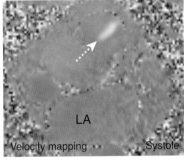

Figure 7.2 *Preoperative CMR assessment of a 73-year-old woman with PS.
(a) Modified sagittal SSFP cine view showing the stenotic pulmonary valve (PV; black arrow), an aneurysmal LPA (maximal diameter 4.2 cm) and right ventricular hypertrophy (RVH). Turbulent blood flow above the valve is noted as signal loss within the otherwise high intensity blood signal. A perpendicular imaging plane was then acquired just above the valve, within the narrow part of the jet (black line). (b) Resulting SSFP cine showing the PV with restricted opening (solid white arrow). (c) Subsequent velocity mapping CMR in the same plane. Peak velocity was measured at 2.8 m/s within the area indicated (dashed white arrow).*

■ CMR in specific ACHD

Congenital heart disease is usually recognized in childhood and the most frequent use of CMR is in the assessment of patients with an established diagnosis.

Ventricular septal defect

VSDs are the most common congenital heart defects. They range from small haemodynamically insignificant and isolated lesions to large defects associated with multiple cardiac anomalies such as in TOF. CMR is complementary to echocardiography in the assessment of simple and complex VSDs. It allows multiplanar visualization of the spatial relationship of the defect to surrounding structures, can diagnose concurrent cardiac pathology and their functional sequelae, and quantify shunt size and effect on the RV and PAs. SE imaging en-face and parallel to the VSD provides anatomical information. SSFP cines show signal loss in the RV due to blood flow through the VSD and are useful in assessing the shape and dimensions of the defect (Figure 7.3). Shunt ratio can be calculated in two ways: firstly, comparison of pulmonary to systemic flow (Qp:Qs) obtained by velocity mapping CMR, and secondly, from the difference in ventricular SV obtained from the ventricular short-axis stack of cines (Figure 7.4).

Specific reporting features in the CMR assessment of VSD are therefore:

1. Description of anatomy;
2. Quantification of shunt size; and
3. Evidence of other cardiac anomalies and consequences, such as complex congenital heart disease and pulmonary hypertension.

Atrial septal defect

There are three types of ASDs, all of which can present initially in adulthood. The commonest defect is the ostium secundum defect (75%) in the area of the foramen ovale. Echocardiography is first line for the diagnosis of ASD. CMR is used where echocardiography is suboptimal, identifying the defect through visualization of low signal on the right side of the atrial septum on SSFP cines. CMR quantifies shunt size, determines the anatomical and functional effects of the shunt, and accurately identifies anomalous pulmonary venous drainage (APVD; Figure 7.5).

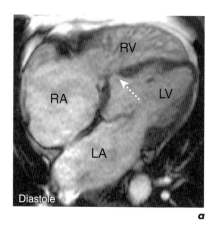 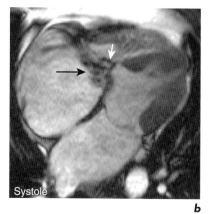

Figure 7.3 *Four-chamber SSFP GE cines from a 65-year-old man with a suspected Gerbode defect (VSD communicating directly between LV and RA).*
(a) *Small, basal, probably muscular VSD is identified (dashed white arrow).* ***(b)*** *Flow through this defect is into the RV (solid white arrow) and not the RA. Associated TR (black arrow) is in fact responsible for the dilated RA. Of note, the apparent interatrial defect seen on these images is a consequence of the imaging plane and not an ASD, and there is RVH.*

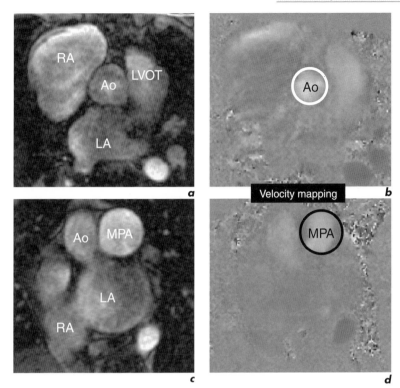

Figure 7.4 *Calculation of Qp:Qs for the VSD case presented in Figure 7.3 using velocity mapping CMR.*
(a, b) Oblique sagittal views of the ascending aorta in cross section by (a) magnitude and (b) phase-subtracted components of velocity mapping CMR. This plane is obtained from the SSFP cine LVOT view by imaging perpendicularly and just distal to the AV. (c, d) Oblique transaxial views of the proximal MPA in cross section by (c) magnitude and (d) phase-subtracted components of velocity mapping CMR. This plane is obtained from the SSFP GE cine RVOT view by imaging perpendicularly and just distal to the PV. (b, d) Flow within the aorta (white circle) and MPA (black circle) is calculated throughout the cardiac cycle and was 5.0 and 9.2 L/min, respectively, giving a Qp:Qs of 1.8:1. Calculations of the Qp:Qs by comparison of SV will be overestimated in the presence of severe TR.

Specific reporting features for ASD are:

1. Description of anatomy including suitability for device closure;
2. Quantification of shunt size; and
3. Evidence of other cardiac anomalies and consequences, such as APVD and pulmonary hypertension.

Partial anomalous pulmonary venous drainage and major aortopulmonary collateral arteries

CMR has a useful role in the detection and serial evaluation of extracardiac venous and arterial vascular anomalies in ACHD, such as partial anomalous pulmonary

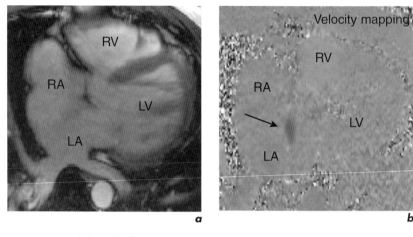

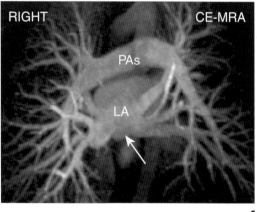

Figure 7.5 *Secundum ASD with Qp:Qs of 2.2:1 calculated by velocity mapping at the aorta and MPA as described with the VSD in Figure 7.4.*
(a) Atrial transaxial SSFP cine used to position the subsequent velocity map. (b) Velocity mapping CMR shows flow from the LA to the RA as signal loss (black arrow). (c) MIP reconstruction of CE-MRA data of the anatomy of the pulmonary vasculature showing no evidence of APVD (white arrow)—there are two right-sided pulmonary veins and three left-sided pulmonary veins.

venous drainage (PAPVD) and major aortopulmonary collateral arteries (MAPCAs). CMR imaging protocols in PAPVD and MAPCAs incorporate MRA for optimal detection of vessels and this often provides additional information to findings at cardiac catheterization as well as confirming the diagnosis (Figure 7.6). Velocity mapping quantifies shunt sizes, and SE techniques can surmount image artefact from endovascular coils.

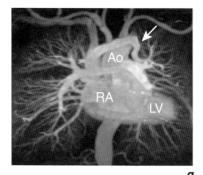
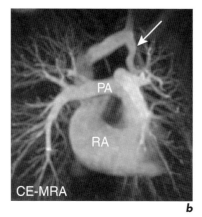

Figure 7.6 *Two MIP reconstructions of CE-MRA data from a 63-year-old woman showing a CMR diagnosis of PAPVD with the left upper pulmonary vein draining via a vertical vein into a dilated left brachiocephalic vein (white arrows).*
Qp:Qs in this case was 1.4:1 and there was no evidence of RV dysfunction or pulmonary hypertension.

CMR reports include:

1. Description of anomalous extracardiac venous or arterial drainage;
2. Quantification of shunt size; and
3. Evidence of other cardiac anomalies and consequences, such as ASD and pulmonary hypertension.

Pulmonary stenosis, right ventricular outflow tract and conduit obstruction

In contrast to the assessment of ASD and VSD, the RVOT and conduits from the RV to the PA are often poorly visualized by echocardiography. CMR provides detailed imaging of the level and anatomy of RVOT obstruction with SE and SSFP cine imaging in orthogonal planes. Serial, contiguous cines in the transaxial plane are useful for functional assessment of extracardiac ventriculopulmonary shunts, such as the Rastelli shunt. Velocity mapping quantifies severity of stenosis or regurgitation and may be used at valve level, within the MPA, or separately within the right and left PAs (Figure 7.7). CE-MRA is an excellent noninvasive method of assessing branch pulmonary stenoses and identification of MAPCAs.

Patent ductus arteriosus and aortopulmonary window

PDA describes persistent arterial communication between the proximal LPA and descending thoracic aorta distal to the origin of the left subclavian artery. It is

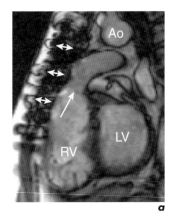
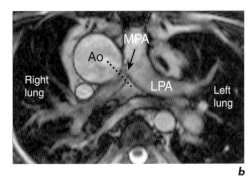

Figure 7.7 *SSFP cines from a 28-year-old man with an underlying diagnosis of truncus arteriosus.*
The patient had undergone the Rastelli procedure (a valved conduit from the anterior wall of the RV to the PA with VSD closure) aged 3. The conduit had been replaced 4 years prior to this CMR study. (a) RVOT view showing the homograft in the pulmonary position to be functioning well without significant stenosis or regurgitation (white arrow). Metallic artefact from sternal wiring is noted (double-headed white arrows). (b) Transaxial view of the MPA and bifurcation into the LPA and RPA shows narrowing at the origin of the latter with relative distal hypoplasia (solid black arrow). Signal loss within the proximal RPA indicates turbulent blood flow and velocity mapping was therefore performed in a plane perpendicular and just distally (dashed black line). Peak velocity was 2.4 m/s, confirming significant proximal RPA stenosis.

usually an isolated lesion in adults. Flow through a PDA is detectable on cines, which show turbulence in the anterior portion of the PA proximal to its bifurcation (Figure 7.8). CMR can quantify shunt size and evaluate signs of pulmonary hypertension prior to decisions regarding device closure.

Aortopulmonary window is a connection between the ascending aorta and PA which presents in a fashion similar to that of PDA and can be differentiated by cines.

Ebstein anomaly

The diagnosis of Ebstein's anomaly is usually made on echocardiography but CMR has a role in defining anatomy and identifying those requiring and suitable for surgical correction (Figure 7.9). Apical displacement of the septal and mural leaflets of the tricuspid valve (TV) is identified on long-axis cines. Serial short-axis cines assess enlargement of the anterior leaflet and degree of TV dysplasia, and are later analysed to provide volumetric and functional data on the RA and RV. Velocity mapping CMR is usually performed in order to quantify the degree of TR, but is occasionally also used to quantify the severity of TS. Both SSFP cines and velocity mapping are used to evaluate the presence of abnormal atrial communication.

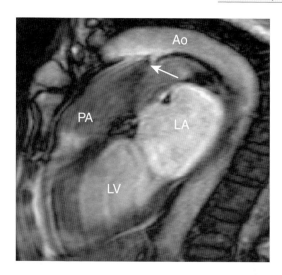

Figure 7.8 *Oblique sagittal SSFP cine view from a 71-year-old woman with Ehlers–Danlos syndrome and PDA (demonstrated by marked signal loss from the aorta into the PA; white arrow).*

Tetralogy of Fallot

TOF comprises VSD, RVOT obstruction, RVH and an overriding aorta. Definitive repair includes VSD patch closure and resection of RVOT obstruction, with older patients often having prior palliative shunt procedures such as the Blalock–Taussig (subclavian to PA anastomosis) shunt. Reconstruction of the RVOT leads to important PR and serial assessments of regurgitation and the RV are crucial following repair. Other postoperative complications, such as aneurysm formation in the RVOT and dilatation of the aortic root, as well as co-existing congenital anomalies, including right-sided aortic arch and aberrant coronary anatomy, can often be identified at the initial orthogonal multi-slice FSE sequences and are then further characterized with higher resolution SSFP sequences.

Serial, contiguous ventricular short-axis cines enable calculation of standard biventricular parameters and also highlight residual septal defects, confirmed using velocity mapping CMR. Comparison of RV and LVSV or velocity mapping above the pulmonary valve (PV) provides PV regurgitant fraction, with a value of 40% representing free PR. Cines and velocity mapping at the RVOT, LPA and RPA evaluate stenoses at these sites. Branch PS can arise due to distortion from palliative arterial shunts, particularly the Pott (descending aorta to LPA) or Waterson (ascending aorta to MPA or RPA) shunts, and may provoke worse PR. Patency of residual shunts should be assessed due to the risk of pulmonary hypertension through augmented pulmonary blood flow.

PREOPERATIVE   POSTOPERATIVE

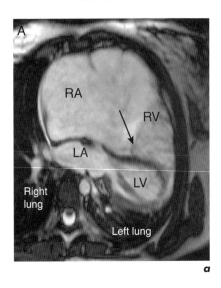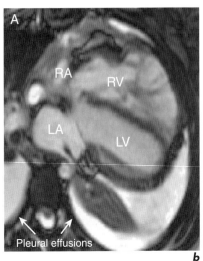

a   *b*

Figure 7.9 *Pre- and postoperative four-chamber SSFP cines from a CMR study performed on a 16-year-old girl with severe Ebstein anomaly.*
(a) There is 4 cm apical displacement of the septal leaflet of the TV (black arrow). The RA, atrialized part of the RV, and RV are dilated. RVEF was 45% in the presence of severe TR, regurgitant fraction 49% by comparison of LV and RVSV. (b) Satisfactory early (day 8) postoperative findings at CMR. Surgery comprised repair of the TV, plication of the RV, cryoablation of the RA, and ASD closure with a fenestrated patch and one-way Gortex flap to allow right-to-left shunting in the presence of elevated RA pressures. The reconstructed TV was noted to be functioning well without TR and only mild tricuspid stenosis (TS), orifice area 3 cm² and peak recorded diastolic velocity of 1.2 m/s.

LGE in the RV and LV is common following TOF repair and is related to adverse clinical markers including ventricular dysfunction. In particular, RV enhancement predicts arrhythmia which has potential prognostic implications (Figure 7.10).

Serial CMR assessments without contrast can be used to monitor drug treatment and determine timing of repeat intervention to the PV.

Specific comments in TOF CMR reports include:

1. Anatomical and functional evaluation of prior interventions (surgical repair and palliative shunts);
2. Quantification of PR (and AR if present);
3. Description of associated congenital anomalies; and
4. Presence and pattern of late enhancement.

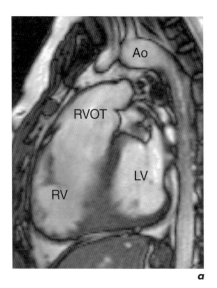 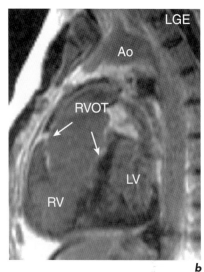

a   b

Figure 7.10 **(a)** RVOT SSFP cine view and **(b)** equivalent LGE view from a 27-year-old man with repaired TOF highlighting areas of enhancement at the free wall and septal surface of the RV (white arrows).

Corrected transposition of the great arteries

In transposition of the great arteries (TGA) the aorta arises from the RV and the PA arises from the LV. Almost all surviving adults with TGA have undergone operative correction in childhood, either removal of the atrial septum and insertion of a baffle (Mustard operation) or folding of the atrial wall (Senning operation), to redirect atrial flow but leaving the transposed ventriculoarterial connections. The primary aim in postoperative imaging is assessment of pulmonary and systemic venous flow pathways (Figure 7.11). CMR readily identifies stenoses and baffle leaks with subsequent multiplanar and multislice evaluation allowing anatomical clarification and accurate quantification. SSFP cines are acquired to visualize each pathway in order to identify narrowing or signal loss due to turbulence. Through-plane velocity mapping is then used to identify flow velocities above 1 m/s, indicative of flow obstruction at atrial level. Dilatation of the azygous and hemi-azygous veins is a useful pointer to significant systemic venous pathway obstruction.

Cine assessment of systemic RV function is very important in these patients since they are at risk of RV failure and TR and AR should be quantified when present.

Late enhancement of the systemic RV is also common in adults after the Mustard or Senning procedures, and the extent correlates with ventricular dysfunction and arrhythmia.

Patients who have undergone corrective arterial switch operations require assessment of supravalvular PS or AS and branch PA stenoses. Such patients are also

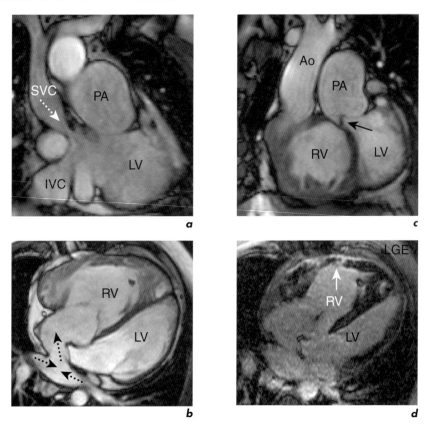

Figure 7.11 *Part of the CMR evaluation in a 30-year-old man who had undergone a Mustard operation for TGA aged 2 months.*
(a) SSFP cine views of the systemic venous pathway shows a narrowed superior vena cava channel (SVC; dashed white arrow) and unobstructed IVC channel. Peak velocities of the two channels were subsequently measured at 1.2 and 1 m/s respectively by velocity mapping CMR. (b) SSFP cine view of the pulmonary venous pathways shows them to be unobstructed (dashed black arrows). (c) SSFP cine view of the outflow tracts reveals RVH and PR (solid black arrow). (d) LGE is noted at the RV free wall (solid white arrow).

at risk of ostial coronary artery stenoses at the site of coronary artery reimplantation, and these can also be evaluated by CMR.

In congenitally corrected transposition of the great arteries (ccTGA), the atria have normal position and venous return but there is atrioventricular discordance together with TGA. CMR identifies the morphological features of each atrium and ventricle, cardiac malposition, and associated congenital anomalies such as VSD, PS or subvalvular PS, and Ebstein-like TV. Accurate functional assessment of the systemic RV, which is susceptible to failure, is required prior to consideration for double switch repairs (Senning and arterial switch).

CMR reports therefore include:

1. Anatomical and functional evaluation of pulmonary and systemic venous flow pathways;
2. Quantification of TR (and AR if present);
3. Description of associated congenital or iatrogenic cardiac abnormalities; and
4. Presence and pattern of LGE.

Univentricular hearts and Fontan repair

In patients with one effective ventricle, the Fontan operation routes systemic venous return directly into the PAs leaving the ventricle to pump oxygenated blood to the systemic circulation. Pulmonary blood flow is dependent on elevated pressure within the systemic veins and any obstruction to flow, such as with thrombus, makes the circuit fail. Contemporary repair involves total cavopulmonary connection, usually by an atrial tunnel or extracardiac conduit. CMR is invaluable in the assessment of such shunts since echocardiography is often limited by the retrosternal position of the connection. Targeted SSFP cines of the connection identify obstruction as signal loss from turbulent blood flow. These acquisitions are also early indicators of RA thrombus formation, which should later be confirmed or refuted using EGE (Figure 7.12). Cine imaging is extended to the pulmonary veins to exclude post-operative compression, with through-plane flow velocities above 1 m/s coinciding with atrial systole being suggestive of obstruction. Serial, contiguous short-axis SSFP cines allow determination of univentricular function and since only one SV value is available, quantification of atrioventricular valve regurgitation requires velocity mapping at the aorta and MPA.

Specific CMR reporting comments for the Fontan circuit are on:

1. Evaluation of the caval pathways, RA, atriopulmonary connection and PAs;
2. Active exclusion of RA thrombus;
3. Evidence of pulmonary venous compression; and
4. Quantification of atrioventricular valve regurgitation.

■ Indications

CMR can:

1. Diagnose, evaluate and safely follow up complex congenital cardiovascular pathology which often spares diagnostic invasive catheterization;
2. Provide highly reproducible imaging for accurate serial assessments including RV function;
3. Diagnose and provide additional information on PAPVD and MAPCAs;
4. Assess the PV and accurately quantify regurgitation and stenoses;
5. Evaluate the PAs and pulmonary veins; and
6. Identify extracardiac and intracardiac shunt patency.

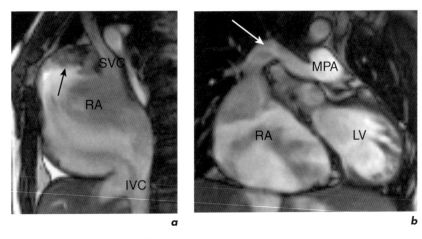

Figure 7.12 *Part of the SSFP GE cine evaluation of a 22-year-old man with a Fontan circuit.*
(a) Assessment of the caval pathways in a near sagittal plane reveals a patent SVC and IVC. The RA is markedly dilated and contains regions of slow flow characterized by signal loss and one area of probable thrombus (black arrow). (b) Assessment of the atriopulmonary connection in a near coronal plane shows a patent conduit from the RA to the MPA (white arrow). Slow flow is once again demonstrated by signal loss within the RA.

CMR cannot:

1. Be used as a screening tool due to limited availability; and
2. Be considered superior to echocardiography for evaluation of most ASDs and simple VSDs.

Chapter 8

Magnetic resonance angiography

Ilse Crevits

■ Introduction

Recent innovations in CMR hardware, such as stronger gradients and faster gradient switching, and software, such as newer pulse sequences and ultrafast MRA techniques, continue to ensure that it is the noninvasive imaging modality of choice in many diseases affecting the great vessels.

Protocols for assessment of the great vessels include low- and high-resolution SE, GE, and ultrafast MRA sequences using gadolinium contrast agent.

■ MRA techniques

Contrast-enhanced MRA

The basic pulse sequence for ultrafast CE-MRA is a 3D GE acquisition which is usually designed to acquire data encoding for contrast first—centric-ordering. The use of gadolinium contrast agent shortens the T1 value of blood so that it appears bright irrespective of flow patterns or velocities (Figure 8.1).

Correct timing of scan acquisition is of paramount importance for optimal imaging of the passage of contrast through the blood vessel of interest. This is usually achieved by application of 'bolus-track' techniques, i.e. a real-time 2D fluoroscopic sequence visualizing the arrival and passage of contrast in the great vessels, which subsequently trigger the high-resolution 3D CE-MRA sequence. The time delay in switching between these two sequences must also be taken into account. Alternative timing methods are the use of a test bolus in order to calculate bolus arrival time, or obtaining a series of ultrashort acquisitions so that at least one acquisition coincides with bolus arrival time.

Time-of-flight (2D or 3D)

This is an older GE technique in which flow signal is enhanced by inflow effects. Stationary tissue within a region of interest is saturated by rapid application of RF pulses. This results in fresh blood flowing into this plane being non-saturated and

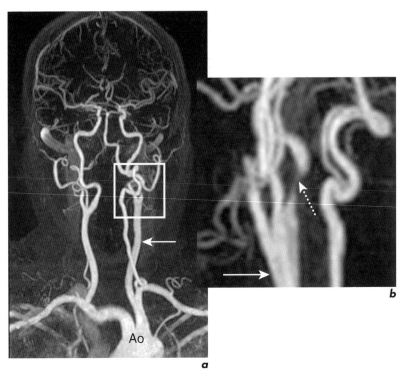

Figure 8.1 *Carotid CE-MRA.*
(a) MIP reconstruction of the entire CE-MRA data. The left common carotid artery (solid white arrow) is seen to have a stenosis following its bifurcation (white square). (b) Enlarged and rotated view of the initial MIP highlights a severe, discrete stenosis at the left internal carotid artery (dashed white arrow).

therefore appearing bright. Unwanted venous signal can be eliminated by application of specific saturation bands. Time-of-flight methods are sensitive to flow velocity; for example, slow flow near the vessel wall appears less bright with this technique than faster flow in the middle of the vessel. Importantly, the 2D time-of-flight sequence has the disadvantage of overestimating vessel stenosis due to a phenomenon known as phase dispersion. This effect is less pronounced using 3D time-of-flight imaging.

■ Post-processing methods

Post-processing algorithms are used to create 3D images. However, they must always be interpreted together with the source images, the 'raw data', to avoid misinterpretation from post-processing induced artefacts (Figure 8.2).

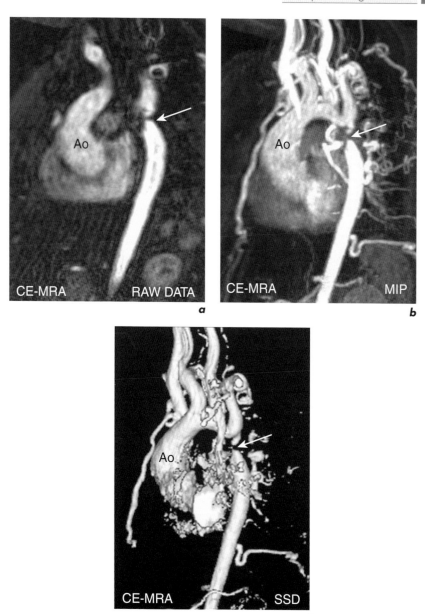

Figure 8.2 *CE-MRA of coarctation of the aorta (white arrows).*
(a) The raw data show a severe narrowing, but this is overestimated in the subsequent
(b) MIP and (c) shaded surface display (SSD) representations. Multiple collaterals are seen
on the MIP and SSD.

Maximal intensity projection

In this ray tracing post-processing algorithm, the desired viewing plane is specified first. Then the maximum intensity encountered in parallel rays along this viewing plane is assigned to the displayed pixel. MIP reconstructions are applicable to both time-of-flight and CE-MRA data and have the tendency to overestimate the degree of vessel stenosis (Figure 8.2b).

Volume rendering technique and shaded surface display

This is a ray casting algorithm which selects visible voxels by tracing rays from an instantaneous viewing position. The surfaces are identified by a threshold technique and the resulting SSD provides 3D appreciation of the vessel. Resulting images can also overestimate the degree of vessel stenosis (Figure 8.2c).

Curved multiplanar reconstruction

Curved multiplanar reconstruction (MPR) can be used to obtain images in views other than that of the native acquisition (Figure 9.3). These work particularly well on 3D data sets with isotropic voxels in which resolution is identical in any obtained plane.

■ Specific Sites

Carotid arteries

The most commonly used sequences for carotid MRA are time-of-flight and CE-MRA (Figure 8.1). For imaging of the aortic arch and cervical arteries, CE-MRA is the only option. Both 3D TOF and CE-MRA are as accurate as conventional X-ray angiography in the measurement of internal carotid artery stenosis, and because of the small but significant risk of stroke with the invasive technique (0.5–1.0%), CMR is recommended as the optimal method of evaluating carotid artery disease. Data interpretation requires careful evaluation of the raw data to avoid overestimation of stenosis severity. MIP projections will aggravate signal loss and cause vessels to appear narrower because the algorithm selects brightest intensities both within the vessel and in the background. Such overestimation with MIPs is more of a problem in 3D time-of-flight than with CE-MRA, in which background intensities are suppressed.

MRA is excellent for the diagnosis of carotid dissection. Dissection typically consists of haemorrhage in the media, sometimes extending into the adventitia, and the intimal flap is not always apparent. Angiography identifies a smooth or irregular narrowing and high-resolution SE images with fat saturation prepulse can help to identify the false lumen.

CE-MRA can also visualize stenoses within the vertebral artery or within the basilar artery. Reversal of blood flow in the vertebral artery with subclavian steal phenomenon is recognized using CE-MRA in combination with through-plane velocity mapping CMR (after handgrip exercise) at the level of the vertebral arteries. Confirmation is with 2D time-of-flight MRA acquired first with an inferior and then a superior saturation band to confirm flow reversal.

Carotid MRA reports concentrate on:

1. Description of internal carotid artery stenoses; their location from the bifurcation, severity and length;
2. Evaluation of concurrent vertebral disease; and
3. Assessment of the aorta arch vessel anatomy and, where relevant, atheroma burden.

Pulmonary vessels

Pulmonary arteries

CMR is well suited for the evaluation of PA anatomy and this is widely used in patients with ACHD where evaluation of the size, patency and anatomical relations of the PAs is combined with RV assessment and PV status. It is also being increasingly used in the assessment of patients with pulmonary hypertension (Figure 8.3). CT pulmonary angiography remains the imaging modality of choice for diagnosis of acute pulmonary embolism since MRA has longer acquisition, and thus breath-hold times, and lower spatial resolution leading to smaller peripheral emboli potentially going undetected.

Pulmonary veins

The use of CMR in the diagnosis and differentiation of the various forms of partial and total APVD has already been discussed. Additionally, it has a role in the evaluation of the pulmonary veins and LA pre-radiofrequency ablation for cardiac arrhythmias. Subsequent assessment of pulmonary vein stenosis requires CE-MRA combined with velocity mapping (Figure 8.4).

The pulmonary veins should also be imaged using CE-MRA in cases of cardiac malignancy involving the LA in order to exclude extension.

MRA reports of the pulmonary vessels include:

1. Description of the anatomy;
2. Concurrent cardiac assessment, such as the RV in ACHD and pulmonary hypertension; and
3. Measurements of pulmonary vein anatomy and orifice diameters in patients referred for radiofrequency ablation.

Renal and mesenteric arteries

CE-MRA is a good method for assessment of the renal arteries, especially in cases of renovascular hypertension due to atherosclerosis and, to a lesser extent, suspected fibromuscular dysplasia.

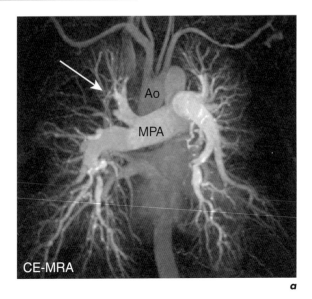

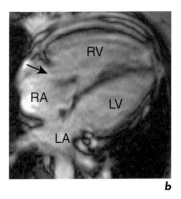

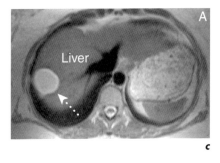

Figure 8.3 *CMR assessment in a 59-year-old woman with pulmonary hypertension secondary to chronic thromboembolic disease.* **(a)** *MIP reconstruction of PA CE-MRA highlighting proximal obstruction of the right upper and middle lobe arteries (solid white arrow). There was also evidence of multiple distal stenoses predominantly in the lower lobe branches.* **(b)** *Concurrent serial SSFP cine cardiac assessment revealed a dilated RV with reduced EF (34%) and moderate TR (black arrow).* **(c)** *An incidental liver cyst seen on the pilot transaxial FSE images (dashed white arrow).*

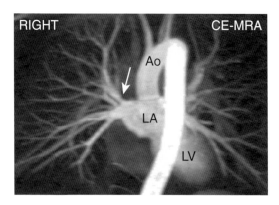

Figure 8.4 *MIP reconstruction of CE-MRA data from a 47-year-old man showing moderate stenosis (50%) of the right upper anterior pulmonary vein following radiofrequency ablation (white arrow).*

CMR screening protocols for secondary causes of hypertension conclude with angiography and are performed during an hour-long study in the following manner:

- Cardiac assessment and later calculation of LV volumes, function and mass;
- Exclusion of coarctation of the aorta;
- Evaluation of the adrenal glands; and
- Renal CE-MRA (Figure 8.5).

CE-MRA provides reliable visualization of the major renal arteries and accessory renal arteries along their entire length. However, spatial resolution remains lower than with conventional X-ray angiography, so branch vessels and small accessory vessels are less well depicted. This is of relevance, for example, in some cases of fibromuscular dysplasia where the main renal arteries may not be involved but smaller side branches are affected. Fibromuscular dysplasia is a much less common cause of renal artery stenosis than atherosclerosis. It principally affects young women who present with hypertension and biochemical abnormalities, but rarely renal impairment. Lesions typically affect the main renal artery, are unilateral, beaded in appearance, and may have multiple stenoses. By comparison, atheromatous renal artery stenosis has a predilection for an older, male population with evidence of atheroma elsewhere, treatment-resistant hypertension, and associated renal dysfunction. Importantly, gadolinium contrast agent is not nephrotoxic. The commonest site for atheromatous renal artery stenosis is at the ostium of the renal artery and multiple lesions affecting different-sized vessels may co-exist. Grading of stenosis severity is assisted by post-processing MPR reconstruction and velocity mapping CMR.

Published data related to mesenteric CE-MRA is limited. Anecdotally, results appear comparable to renal angiography. Most stenoses in the coeliac trunk and superior mesenteric artery occur within the proximal segment where the diameter of

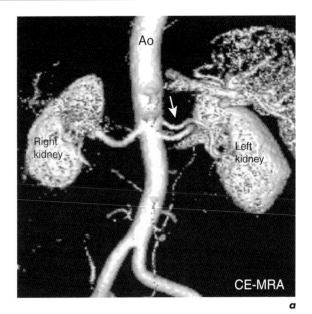

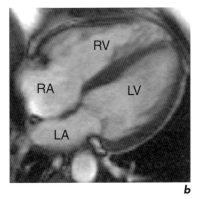

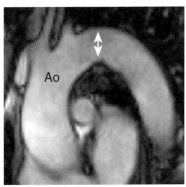

Figure 8.5 *Part of a CMR hypertension screen from a 55-year-old man.*
(a) SSD reconstruction of the renal CE-MRA data showing no evidence of renal artery stenosis. A left accessory renal artery is indicated (white arrow). (b) Prior serial SSFP GE cine cardiac assessment was later analysed to reveal normal LV size, volume and function, with mild LVH. (c) Oblique sagittal SSFP GE cine image showing no evidence of coarctation of the aorta (two-headed white arrow).
High-resolution T1W SE images of the adrenal glands were normal and are not illustrated in this figure.

the vessel is the greatest. The inferior mesenteric artery is often less well visualized since it is smaller and consequently stenoses at this site are often overestimated by CMR.

Renal MRA reports include:

1. Description of renal anatomy, such as kidney size and cortical architecture;
2. Description of renal arteries and stenoses when present;
3. Additional comments on LV mass and function, exclusion of coarctation of the aorta, and presence of adrenal pathology in cases of hypertension screening.

Aorta

The thoracic aorta has already been discussed in Chapter 6. Optimal visualization of the aorta is via a combination of SE and GE techniques to ensure accurate evaluation of the aortic wall and peri-aortic tissues, and lumen, respectively. With inflammatory conditions, such as aortitis, contrast agents are used to further highlight aortic wall abnormalities. CE-MRA readily depicts location, extent and exact diameter of aortic aneurysms with measurements being made on the original images (Figure 8.6). In cases of aortic dissection where there is continuation to the abdominal aorta it is important to know whether side branches originate from the true or false lumen. CT is often the modality of choice for investigating acute pathology of the aorta, for reasons of both safety and availability, while CMR is an ideal method for patient follow-up following surgical or medical treatment.

MRA reports on the abdominal aorta include:

1. Description of anatomy and likely aetiology of aneurysmal dilatation where present;
2. Evidence of intramural thrombus or dissection; and
3. Proximity to and involvement of key branch vessels in any pathology, such as the renal and iliac arteries.

Peripheral arteries

CE-MRA is the best CMR technique for evaluating arterial disease in the upper and lower limbs. Visualization of the subclavian and brachial arteries requires a dedicated body coil, otherwise the technique is similar to that of thoracic aorta MRA. In order to avoid venous overlap the contrast should be injected in the contralateral arm. Imaging of the small arteries of the hand requires high-resolution scanning, dedicated surface coils, and precise timing of the start of imaging. An additional use of CE-MRA is in the diagnosis of thoracic outlet syndrome where images are acquired with the arms in abduction and in neutral position (Figure 8.7). High-resolution targeted T1W SE sequences are required to demonstrate the cause of compression in this condition.

For imaging of the lower limbs, the most commonly used technique is the bolus chase technique. With this, the first step is the production of mask images of all three stations of the leg: aortoiliac region, femoral region and lower legs. Then, during

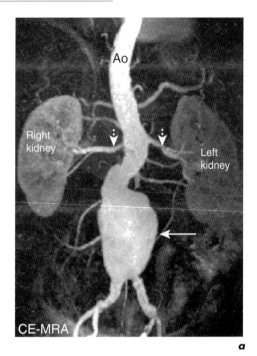

a

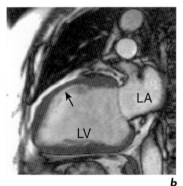

b

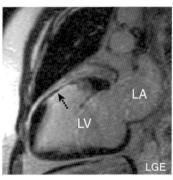

c

Figure 8.6 *CMR study from a 62-year-old man referred prior to elective CABG for further investigation of chronic renal failure.*

(a) MIP reconstruction of CE-MRA data showing a diffusely atherosclerotic abdominal aorta with a large (6.4 × 7.0 × 8.7 cm³) infra-renal aneurysm (solid white arrow). The aneurysmal segment starts 4.0 cm after the origin of the renal arteries and has a proximal neck measuring 2.5 cm in diameter. The common iliac arteries arise from the distal aspect of the dilatation. Multilayered mural thrombus was noted within the aneurysm on SE imaging (images not shown). The right and left renal arteries had only mild stenoses (dashed white arrow) and the kidneys are of comparable size. (b) Part of the prior SSFP GE cine assessment demonstrating thinning of the mid-anterior wall on the two-chamber view (solid black arrow). (c) This segment was associated with near transmural late enhancement indicative of MI and non-viable myocardium (dashed black arrow).

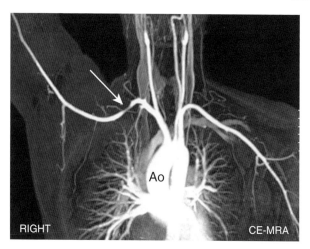

Figure 8.7 *MIP reconstruction of CE-MRA data from a 30-year-old woman with thoracic outlet syndrome.*
Images were acquired with the right arm in elevation and abduction (symptomatic position) and show a stenosis in the proximal subclavian artery (white arrow). CE-MRA with the arm in neutral position did not reveal any abnormalities (not shown).

constant injection of contrast, the contrast bolus is followed throughout the entire leg using a moving table. Imaging of the tibial vessels may be compromised by venous contamination. Steno-occlusive disease in the distal aorta is readily seen as in Leriche's syndrome and CE-MRA is also useful in the surveillance of extra-anatomical bypass grafts (Figure 8.8).

■ Indications

MRA can:

1. Diagnose internal carotid artery stenoses as well as conventional X-ray angiography without the small but significant risk of stroke. It has an important role in the preoperative evaluation of carotid artery disease prior to cardiac and vascular surgery;
2. Readily provide information on the anatomical relationships, size and patency of pulmonary arteries and veins. This gives CMR a useful role in ACHD, pulmonary hypertension, and pre- and post-radiofrequency ablation;
3. Evaluate the renal and mesenteric arteries;
4. Screen for secondary causes of hypertension;
5. Assess congenital and acquired aortic disease;
6. Be used at a variety of peripheral arterial sites for the assessment of suspected atherosclerotic occlusive disease; and
7. Provide safe, serial patient follow-up.

MRA cannot:

1. Be considered first line in haemodynamically unstable patients; and
2. Be used in preference to CT for suspected pulmonary embolism.

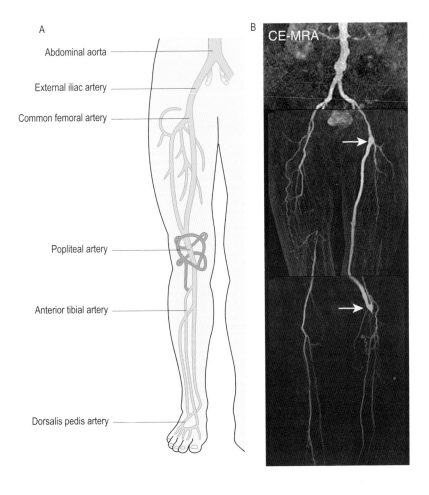

Figure 8.8 *Lower limb CE-MRA.*
(a) Diagrammatic representation of normal lower limb arterial anatomy. (b) MIP reconstruction of CE-MRA data from a 70-year-old man presenting with intermittent claudication on a background of a left femoropopliteal bypass graft operation. The graft is shown to be patent (between white arrows).

Chapter 9

Coronary MRA

Anitha Varghese

■ Introduction

Coronary MRA is technically demanding since the coronary arteries are small, tortuous vessels embedded in epicardial fat that move with cardiac and respiratory motion.

> The current clinical utility of coronary CMR is limited to visualization of proximal coronary artery anatomy, predominantly for the diagnosis of anomalous coronary arteries for which CMR is a class I indication.

■ Coronary MRA techniques

Available techniques are free breathing or breath-hold. These can provide either 2D or 3D data sets using SE or GE sequences. For clinical imaging, we recommend using 3D free breathing or breath-hold SSFP GE techniques. In both methods, scans are ECG-gated to commence at mid to late diastole when cardiac motion is minimal. Optimal fat suppression is mandatory. Gadolinium contrast agent is not routinely given.

Free breathing combined with 3D imaging provides good signal-to-noise ratio (SNR) and anatomical coverage. GE sequences image blood within the coronaries, and SE sequences image the vessel wall. Subjects breathe normally throughout the scan and respiratory artefact is minimized by the prior addition of *respiratory navigators*. These provide a way of monitoring respiratory motion during data collection and correcting that data for the motion. Methods of motion assessment differ, and one commonly used is detection of the superior–inferior movement of the dome of the right hemidiaphragm (Figure 9.1). Following placement and navigator initiation, the user automatically accepts data when the diaphragm–lung interface falls within a predefined window and rejects data that fall outside this narrow limit. The acceptance window is positioned at the end expiratory pause period of the respiratory cycle and extends 2–3 mm either side of a patient-specific diaphragm–lung interface value.

Free breathing sequences acquire data over several minutes and provide higher resolution than breath-hold techniques. Breath-hold 3D GE coronary MRA requires subjects to suspend their respiration for 20–25 s depending on their heart rate. Since navigators are avoided, breath-holding requires less expertise and circumvents problems arising from suboptimal respiratory patterns. The resolution and coverage sacrificed with the breath-hold option becomes relevant at the limits of coronary MRA indications, such as evaluation of coronary artery stenoses, and

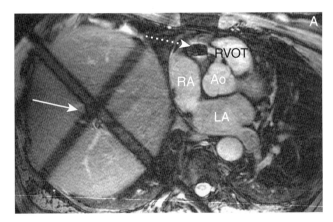

Figure 9.1 *3D free breathing GE coronary MRA sequence in an oblique transaxial plane showing characteristic signal loss from the respiratory navigator on the dome of the right hemidiaphragm (solid white arrow) and a RCA stent (dashed white arrow).*

is not of significance for delineation of proximal coronary artery origin and early course. With free breathing SSFP GE coronary MRA a typical spatial resolution is $1.1 \times 0.7 \times 1.5\,mm^3$ with 30 to 48 mm through-plane coverage, as compared to $1.3 \times 1.1 \times 1.6\,mm^3$ with 16 to 19.2 mm through-plane coverage using the breath-hold sequence. Breath-holding permits several volumes of interest to be imaged in the same time it takes to perform one free breathing scan. Patients do vary in their response to the two methods with consequent compromise to image quality and diagnostic accuracy, and both may need to be attempted (Figure 9.2). Maximal and optimal resolution with either technique is not equivalent. Maximizing resolution will assist accuracy but will reduce SNR and lead to grainy images, while optimal resolution may be a little lower but produce better quality scans. Post-processing curved MPR is an excellent way of presenting findings in coronary MRA reports (Figure 9.3).

■ Coronary MRA protocol

Coronary MRA protocols for evaluation of proximal coronary artery origins and course take approximately 15 to 20 min to perform:

- Initial pilot FSE acquisitions are obtained in the three orthogonal planes: transaxial, coronal and sagittal. This usually results in localization of at least one of the coronary artery origins from the aortic root (Figure 9.4).
- Oblique transaxial 3D imaging volumes are then acquired around this region either with or without the addition of a respiratory navigator depending on user preference.
- Further acquisitions are planned from these images. Successive oblique transaxial views tend to be the most easy to interpret, and more than one plane is required to interrogate ostial narrowing.

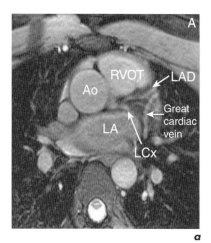
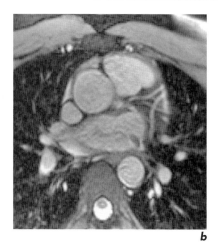

a

b

Figure 9.2 *Raw data MRA of the left coronary system from a normal 32-year-old male subject in an oblique transaxial plane demonstrating equivalent image quality using **(a)** free breathing and **(b)** breath-hold techniques. With kind permission from Varghese, Keegan and Pennell, Coronary Artery Dis, P. 2005; 16: 355–364.*

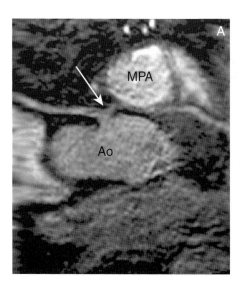

Figure 9.3 *Curved MPR showing the rare, interarterial left main stem (LMS) anomaly originating from the right sinus of Valsalva (SoV; white arrow). This variant is considered the highest risk for ischaemia and sudden death.*

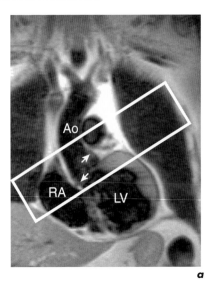 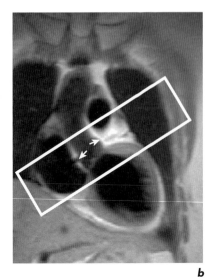

a   *b*

Figure 9.4 *Two examples of pilot coronal FSE imaging showing approximate coronary artery origins from the aortic root (white arrows). Subsequent high-resolution 3D coronary MRA data acquisition is targeted to a volume of interest centred in an oblique transaxial plane encompassing these origins (white rectangle).*

- Poor quality images should result in:
  - switching techniques (free breathing/breath-hold);
  - double checking that fat suppression has been optimized; and
  - reiterating relevant patient instructions. For free breathing methods patients are asked to relax and breathe normally, while breath-holding may need to be tried at maximal inspiration rather than expiration. End expiratory respiratory positions are more reproducible and prone to less diaphragmatic drift, however, end inspiration may be better tolerated.
- Functional consequences of malignant anomalies are evaluated with perfusion CMR (Chapter 2).

■ Anomalous coronary arteries

Anomalous coronary arteries are rare and usually asymptomatic. Prevalence ranges from 1% in patients with otherwise normal cardiac anatomy to 36% in individuals with ACHD such as TOF. Their importance lies in the association of specific variants with myocardial ischaemia or MI, syncope and sudden cardiac death, particularly amongst young adults. This premature morbidity and mortality typically occurs during strenuous physical exercise with coronary arteries that traverse between the aorta and PA (Figure 9.3). Three postulated mechanisms are: mechanical embarrassment from aortic and PA dilatation at a time of increased coronary flow demand, kinking of an ostial or proximal segment due to a sharp turn or bend at the origin, and a congenitally slit-like ostium which is inadequate to meet extra requirements.

Variations of anomalies include:

- Origin of the LCx from the right SoV or RCA (Figure 9.5)—this accounts for greater than 50% of cases, usually with a benign course behind the aorta (retroaortic);
- Origin of the RCA from the left SoV—this accounts for 20–25% of cases, usually with a course between the PA/proximal RVOT and aorta (interarterial); and
- Rarely, origin of the LMS or LAD from the right SoV with an interarterial course. Alternative proximal pathways for these vessels are retroaortic, anterior to the PA, and intraseptal.

Coronary MRA is less helpful in the direct visualization of fistulas and coronary origination outside the sinuses of Valsalva, such as from the PAs.

Referrals for coronary MRA are often made following X-ray coronary angiography where there is failure to engage one of the coronary ostia, or when an anomaly is angiographically demonstrated and delineation of the proximal course is needed. Coronary MRA is important in patients with ACHD and as part of the work-up in young patients with unexplained syncope or chest pain. These latter groups invariably undergo more comprehensive CMR evaluation than coronary MRA alone. A potential preparticipation screening role in competitive athletes has also been

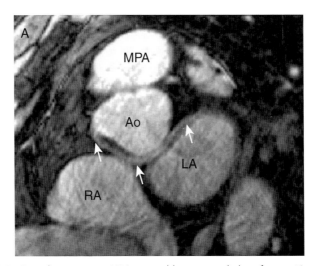

Figure 9.5 *Raw data coronary MRA in an oblique sagittal plane from a 63-year-old male patient with hypertension and a positive exercise tolerance test.*
X-ray coronary angiography revealed a non-dominant RCA, patent LAD and aberrant LCx arising from the right SoV. Coronary MRA was requested in order to evaluate the course of the LCx, which is seen to be the common retroaortic variant (white arrows).

suggested, again with a CMR protocol encompassing more than isolated exclusion of anomalous coronary arteries.

Clinical reports comment on:

1. Presence or absence of anomalous origins and ostial appearance;
2. Subsequent coronary artery course;
3. Length of total artery adequately visualized; and
4. Perfusion CMR findings if acquired.

■ Coronary artery aneurysms and Kawasaki disease

Coronary artery aneurysms are rare. Causes are congenital or acquired secondary to atherosclerosis, coronary interventions and connective tissue or inflammatory disorders such as Kawasaki disease (Figure 9.6). Kawasaki disease is a vasculitis affecting children. Cardiovascular complications are the leading cause of mortality and morbidity and include myocarditis and valvular regurgitation. Coronary artery aneurysms can lead to MI, sudden death or IHD and sites for aneurysm formation in reducing order of frequency are:

- Proximal LAD and proximal RCA;
- LMS;
- LCx;
- Distal RCA; and the
- Junction between the RCA and posterior descending coronary artery.

The commonest sites are therefore accessible for coronary MRA, which is usually requested following TTE diagnosis in childhood. Current management guidelines for patients with a solitary, small to medium sized aneurysm (between 3 and 6 mm) in one or more coronary arteries are annual ECG and TTE, and stress testing with myocardial perfusion imaging every 2 years after the age of 10. Patients with at least one large coronary artery aneurysm (≥ 6 mm), or segmented aneurysms without evidence of coronary artery obstruction, and those with evidence of coronary artery obstruction at X-ray angiography, are suggested to have biannual ECG and TTE and annual stress tests with myocardial perfusion evaluation. Additionally, peripheral and abdominal angiography may be required prior to the first X-ray coronary angiography procedure since aneurysms can also occur outside the coronary arterial system. Common sites include the subclavian, femoral and iliac arteries, with less frequent involvement at the abdominal aorta and renal arteries. CMR is therefore an ideal modality for follow-up in this condition.

Clinical reports on cardiac findings comprise:

1. Details on coronary artery aneurysm location and dimensions, and length of artery adequately visualized;
2. Evidence of MR or AR on cine imaging;
3. Exclusion of myocarditis and MI using a combination of cines and LGE; and
4. Perfusion CMR results.

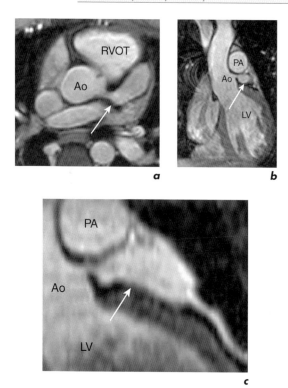

Figure 9.6 *3D breath-hold GE coronary MRA in a 14-year-old boy showing a giant left coronary artery aneurysm (white arrows) secondary to previous Kawasaki disease.*
(a, b) Raw data in oblique transaxial and coronal planes. The aneurysm involved the LMS 5 mm from its ostium with extension into the proximal LAD and dimensions of 33 × 16 mm².
(c) Curved MPR from repeat CMR evaluation performed 8 months later suggested no change in aneurysm size.

■ Indications

Coronary MRA can:

1. Diagnose anomalous coronary arteries; and
2. Be used for surveillance of proximal coronary artery aneurysms.

Coronary MRA cannot:

1. Achieve the resolution of X-ray coronary angiography for the identification and grading of coronary artery stenoses; and
2. Achieve the resolution of CT coronary angiography, nor identify coronary artery calcification.

Chapter 10

Common CMR artefacts

Chad A Hoyt

■ Introduction

CMR can provide excellent static and dynamic images but some knowledge of artefacts is important when unusual findings occur or suboptimal images are obtained.

■ Motion artefact

Patient motion artefacts are common, and are also referred to as *phase mismapping* or *ghosting* (Figure 10.1). Two important reasons for these artefacts are respiratory

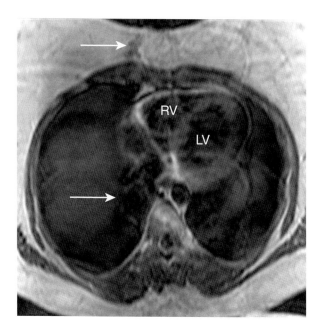

Figure 10.1 *SE images demonstrate ghosting of the cardiac silhouette along the phase encode axis caused by cardiac motion artefact (arrows).*

and cardiac motion. Other causes are flow and actual patient bodily movement on the table. Image distortion is due to anatomical movement between the application of the phase and frequency encoding gradients, leading to within-view errors, and anatomical motion between each application of the phase encoding gradient, causing view-to-view errors. Motion artefacts always occur along the direction of the phase encoding gradient, the phase encode axis, and appear as blurring across an image. Periodic motion will be located at regular intervals along the phase encode axis with the shape of the ghost reflecting the moving structure. The false images usually have increased signal intensity at the expense of the causal moving structure, from which signal is reduced. There are several ways to reduce motion artefact. General measures include swapping the direction of the phase and frequency encoding gradients so that the ghosting falls outside the area of interest, and vendor-specific gradient moment rephasing methods which can automatically correct altered phases back to their original values. More specific measures directed at respiratory and cardiac motion are discussed below.

Respiratory motion

Respiratory motion artefacts are usually eliminated by instructing patients to hold their breath at end expiration throughout the duration of scanner noise (Figure 10.2). If this is unsuccessful, then the operator should firstly reiterate the importance of total suspension of breathing during image acquisition and repeat the scan (Figure 10.3). Following failure of repeated instruction, breath-holding can be tried at maximal inspiration or the scan acquisition time shortened by the addition of *parallel acquisition*. These methods employ computational techniques and arrays of coils wherein each coil independently and simultaneously images a given volume. Parallel imaging can be used to either reduce the total

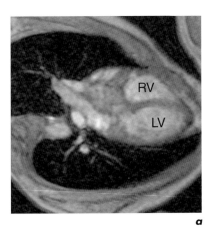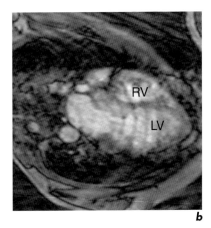

a *b*

Figure 10.2 *GE images* **(a)** *with and* **(b)** *without breath-holding during scan acquisition show blurring induced by movement of the anterior chest wall.*

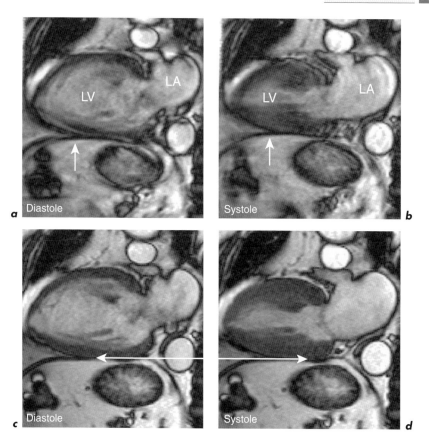

Figure 10.3 *Two-chamber SSFP cine images from a 71-year-old patient with dyspnoea secondary to functional AR resulting from a dilated aortic root and proximal aorta. (**a, b**) Highlight significant upward diaphragmatic motion (white arrows) at the first attempt, which leads to loss of cardiac image clarity. (**c, d**) Repeat imaging after repeat instruction result in no diaphragmatic motion (double-headed white arrow) and are consequently much improved.*

acquisition time or increase the resolution of a scan. There will be some loss of image quality in return for reduced scan duration. Respiratory navigator techniques can also be tried as in coronary MRA. Additionally, a prepulse RF signal can be directed across the chest wall to reduce or eliminate signal coming from it. Such prepulses are either spatially selective or chemically selective. Chemically selective prepulses tend to remove signal from methylene (CH_2) protons in adipose tissue and are therefore means of fat suppression.

Cardiac motion

This is generally reduced using ECG-gating, which synchronizes data acquisition with the phases of the cardiac cycle which are identified relative to the R-R interval.

R-R signal is detected using externally placed ECG electrodes as part of patient preparation for CMR. Problems from inadequate R-R signal necessitate alternative ECG electrode selection, placement, or further patient skin preparation to increase electrode adhesion, while problems with varying R-R interval are more troublesome. This occurs in arrhythmias such as atrial fibrillation, frequent ventricular ectopics, and ventricular bigeminy (Figure 10.4). Atrial fibrillation requires the use of a variation of the ECG-gating process known as *prospective gating*. This is as opposed to *retrospective gating* methods, which acquire data continuously during the cardiac cycle. Retrospective gating is suitable when the R-R interval is regular since the same part of the data is acquired at the same point. When the R-R interval becomes erratic then the shortest interval period is chosen and data are obtained only during that period for each subsequent cycle until the imaging sequence is complete. With frequent ventricular ectopy, a specific arrhythmia rejection program can be instituted to recognize and eliminate the unwanted data. Ventricular bigeminy causes the greatest disruption to image quality and can be counteracted by attempting to exclusively acquire data from the 'normal' cardiac cycles, which will prolong scan duration, or pharmacological methods of arrhythmia suppression such as short-acting prior beta-blocker treatment. Parallel acquisition is also useful for reducing cardiac motion artefacts when used to reduce scan duration.

Summary

Aetiology: Respiratory or cardiac motion, patient movement
Appearance: Ghosting or blurring
Action(s):
Respiratory—Breath-holding, adding respiratory compensation algorithm
Cardiac—Changing ECG lead placement or trying different ECG triggering hardware, prospective versus retrospective gating, arrhythmia rejection software, pharmacological arrhythmia control
Other—Swapping phase and frequency encode axis direction, and parallel acquisition methods for reducing scan duration

■ Metallic artefact

Examples of metallic artefact, or magnetic susceptibility artefact, have been shown throughout this book. A magnetic field is altered by tissues and other materials placed within it. The ability of a material within this field to produce additional magnetism is referred to as *susceptibility*. The susceptibility of water is defined as zero, while air and bone have negative susceptibility since they induce magnetic fields weaker than that of water. Ferromagnetic metals such as iron, and paramagnetic metals such as titanium or nitinol (a titanium alloy), strengthen magnetic fields in their vicinity and are said to have positive susceptibility. Magnetic fields become most heterogeneous near boundaries between substances with different susceptibilities, as in metallic objects within or adjacent to the patient. This heterogeneity alters the precessional frequency of protons and changes their phase (phase incoherence) resulting in artefact.

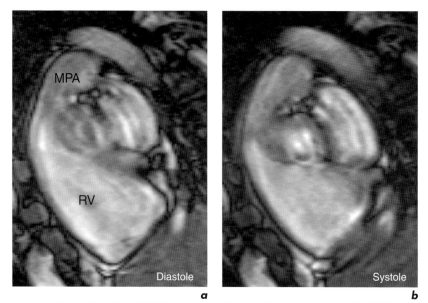

a   *b*

Figure 10.4   *Blurred RVOT SSFP cine frames from a 33-year-old patient with ARVC obtained during an episode of ventricular bigeminy.*

Metallic artefacts on GE sequences appear as varying degrees of signal void and high intensity accompanied by image distortion (Figures 10.5 and 10.6). SE sequences rephase some of the phase incoherence and therefore allow improved imaging (Figure 6.11). Signal void will remain unless the metallic object contains

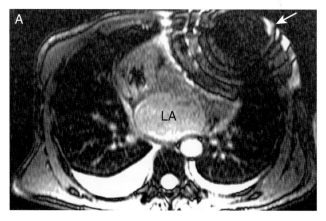

Figure 10.5   *Characteristic metallic artefact (arrowed) on a pilot transaxial GE image secondary to inadvertent imaging of a 58-year-old man with a permanent pacemaker in situ. Permanent pacemakers remain a contraindication to CMR at most centres.*

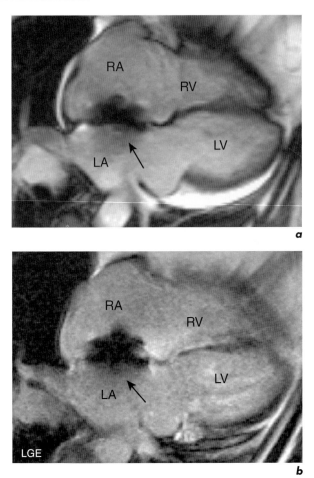

Figure 10.6 *(a)* Cine and *(b)* LGE imaging showing metallic artefact from an Amplatzer ASD closure device (arrowed).

protons, signals from which can be imaged. Whenever possible all metallic items are removed from patients prior to scan initiation.

Summary

Aetiology: Susceptibility differences
Appearance: Signal void, high intensity signal and image distortion
Action: Remove metal if possible, use of SE sequences

■ Wrap-around

This is a common artefact which occurs when the selected field-of-view of imaging is smaller than the anatomical structure being imaged, leading to details outside the area of interest being mapped onto the final image. With modern scanners wrap-around is usually only problematic in the phase encode axis. The appearance is that a structure from position X is mapped into position Y or one side of the image overlaps the other (Figure 10.7). Reduction of wrap can involve increasing the field-of-view, or reducing signal from structures outside the original field-of-view by placement of spatially selective prepulses. Increasing the field-of-view by alterations

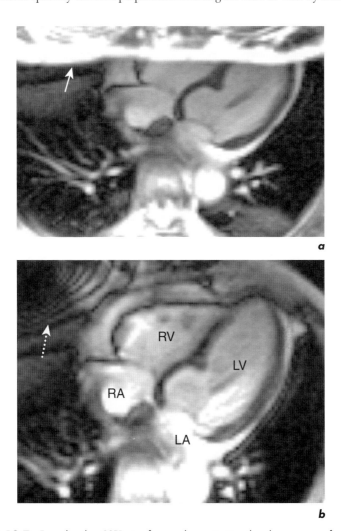

a

b

Figure 10.7 *Four-chamber SSFP cine frames demonstrating the phenomenon of wrap-around (or wrap) in a 62-year-old patient.*
(a) The posterior chest wall has been mapped onto the anterior chest wall (solid white arrow). (b) Increased data acquisition in the phase encode axis eliminates the wrap, lengthens scan duration, and highlights some metallic artefact on the anterior chest wall (dashed white arrow).

to the frequency or phase encode axis can reduce image resolution and increase scan duration respectively. Oversampling of data in the phase encode direction also increases scan time. A certain amount of wrap is acceptable in most clinical imaging as long as there is no ambiguity as to the cause of the artefact, and the area of interest is visualized in full.

> **Summary**
>
> *Aetiology*: Insufficient data sampling
> *Appearance*: Image wrap
> *Action*: Increase field-of-view, oversampling in phase encode axis, foldover suppression in the phase axis
> *Trade-off*: Reduced resolution, prolonging scan duration (this can increase motion artefact)

■ Shimming artefact

Shimming effects are due to magnetic field inhomogeneities. A shim coil can be placed within the area of inhomogeneity to create evenness, a process referred to as *shimming*. Individual patient characteristics will result in bright or dark signal inhomogeneities (Figure 10.8). Most shimming is now automated but can still be performed manually if required in a few minutes (Figure 10.9).

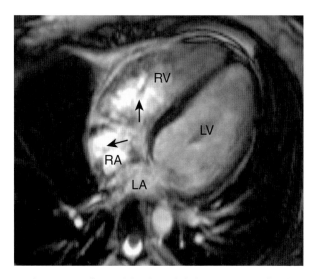

Figure 10.8 *Shimming artefact with bright and dark areas seen within the RA and RV (black arrows) in a patient with liver iron overload from blood transfusions for thalassaemia.*

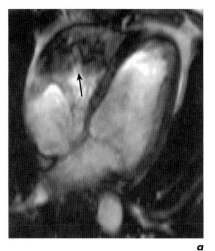 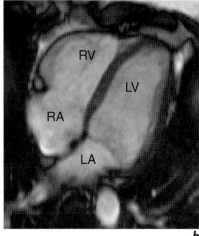

a　　　　　　　　　　　　　　　　　　　　*b*

Figure 10.9 *Beneficial effects of **(a)** pre- and **(b)** post-manual shimming on the clarity and pattern of blood flow within the RV (black arrow) shown on serial four-chamber SSFP cines.*

Summary

Aetiology: Magnetic field inhomogeneities
Appearance: Bright or dark signal
Action: Passive shimming performed by magnet vendor at installation, active or manual shimming performed by operator activating specialized coils

■ Anatomical mimicry

Some routine findings in CMR can appear to represent pathology if not previously encountered, and two important appearances are that of the crista terminalis in the RA and the superior pericardial reflection. The former can be mistaken for a RA mass while the latter can mimic aortic dissection (Figure 10.10).

■ Chemical shift edge artefacts

Protons within fat and water have dissimilar chemical environments and so their precessional frequencies vary; this difference is termed a *frequency shift* and is responsible for chemical shift artefacts. Application of chemically selective prepulses to saturate the signal from fat can improve images in cases of both chemical shift misregistration and cancellation artefact.

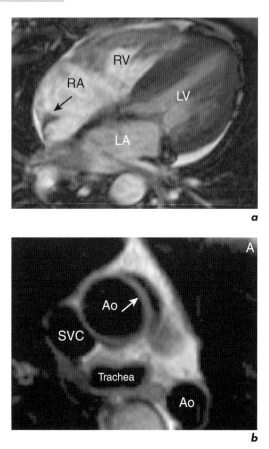

Figure 10.10 **(a)** *Four-chamber SSFP cine frame showing a prominent crista terminalis within the RA (black arrow).* **(b)** *Transaxial FSE demonstrating the superior pericardial reflection adjacent to the ascending aorta (white arrow).*

Chemical shift misregistration

Incorrect mapping of protons with different precessional frequencies leads to signal dis-placement of fat and water along the frequency encode axis which can appear as high signal bands or a signal void between these materials (Figure 10.11). Resulting artefact is proportional to the strength of the magnetic field, with greater frequency shift and therefore artefact noted at higher field strength. Increasing resolution along the frequency encode axis results in the physical distance corresponding to chemical shift artefact being reduced.

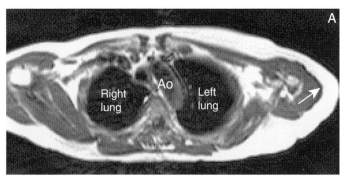

Figure 10.11 *SE image highlighting signal void (chemical shift artefact) along the frequency encode axis at the boundary between subcutaneous fat and water within the left deltoid muscle (white arrow).*

Chemical shift cancellation

When protons within fat and water spin out-of-phase simultaneously, signal intensity is reduced or lost due to signal cancellation. The out-of-phase image produces an asymmetrical edging effect in the phase encode axis and causes a dark ring to form around structures that contain both fat and water. SE sequences use RF rephasing pulses which correct for phase discrepancies and therefore reduce artefact. On GE sequences the echo time parameter can be altered to try to catch the fat and water in-phase, this can lead to a reduction in the number of slices obtained.

■ External artefact

Devices

Artefacts from externally placed devices are usually obvious since they are expected following patient positioning in the magnet. A common example is the ECG box required for obtaining ECG-gated images (Figure 10.12).

Radiofrequency noise

Stripe artefacts along the phase encode axis away from the point of zero frequency encoding can result from extraneous radiofrequency noise, such as radio or television signals (Figure 10.13).

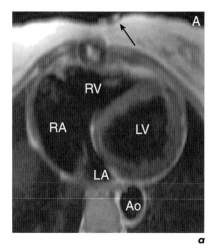

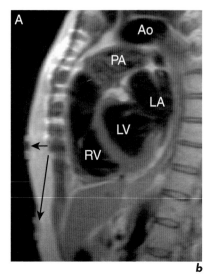

Figure 10.12 *Pilot transaxial and sagittal FSE acquisitions showing external artefact from an ECG box required for obtaining ECG-gated cardiac images (black arrows).*

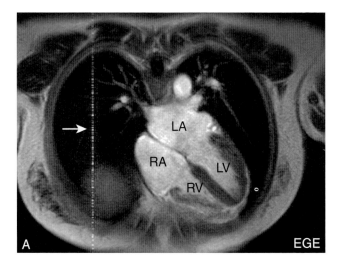

Figure 10.13 *Four-chamber EGE sequence with a single frequency artefact (arrow) caused by the door not being completely closed and allowing extraneous RF noise into the scanner room during image acquisition.*

■ Partial volume effects

Partial volume effects occur due to the finite limits of image resolution. Image resolution is determined by the size of *image voxels*. Within a voxel signals cannot be resolved and an average signal intensity is produced. An increase in resolution is required to obtain smaller voxels, at the expense of SNR. Small or thin structures entirely contained within a voxel may disappear following averaging. This can lead to missing stenosis within coronary arteries by coronary MRA, and poor visualization of thin structures such as valves in certain planes (Figure 10.14).

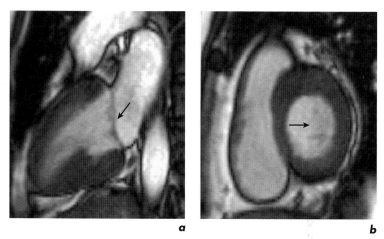

a   *b*

Figure 10.14 *SSFP GE cine frames in the **(a)** two-chamber and **(b)** basal ventricular short-axis views showing the effect of partial voluming on the appearance of the MV (black arrows). Slice thickness is 7 mm for these cines and RF signal solely from the thin MV cannot be differentiated in the latter plane.*

Summary

Aetiology: Structure is entirely contained within a slice
Appearance: Image becomes a combination of structures
Action: Take thinner slices (giving smaller voxels)
Trade-off: Decreased SNR

■ Others

Cross talk

Cross talk occurs as a consequence of interference among adjacent slices. Slice selection profiles are not perfectly rectangular and there is overlap at the edges if they are closely spaced. RF pulses for one slice can then stimulate protons in adjacent slices. Such cross talk often happens in multislice, multiangle acquisitions and gives the appearance of dark bands of signal loss across an image. Insertion of adequate spacing between slices (interslice gap) and obtaining slices in a non-contiguous manner (slice interleaving) both reduce this artefact.

Summary

Aetiology: Slice excitation overlap
Appearance: Dark bands of signal loss
Action: Insertion of interslice gap (minimum 10%), or slice interleaving

Truncation artefacts

Truncation artefacts are also known as ringing, or *Gibbs artefacts*. CMR images are normally the result of image approximation by Fourier transformation. Artefacts arise as a fundamental consequence of the Fourier representation of an image when signal intensity is abrupt and not gradual (gets truncated). Truncation artefacts can be in the frequency or phase encode direction. Truncation can give the appearance of multiple, parallel lines adjacent to high contrast interfaces looking like edge ringing or a syrinx-like stripe (Figure 10.15). False widening of the high contrast interface edges is commonly seen and edge enhancement of the interface with adjacent tissue distortion can also occur. Truncation artefacts can be reduced by increasing the spatial resolution or decreasing the interface contrast. The former can be achieved by sampling for a greater time in the phase encode direction and obtaining a greater number of phase encode steps, while an example of the latter is application of fat suppression for truncation artefact adjacent to adipose tissue.

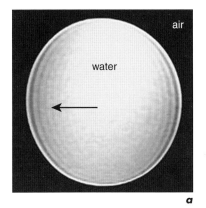 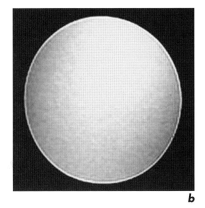

Figure 10.15 *Phantom experiments demonstrating reduction of truncation artefact (black arrow) by increased spatial resolution, in this case doubling the number of phase encode steps obtained from (a) 128 to (b) 256.*

Summary

Aetiology: Abrupt change in image signal intensity
Appearance: Edge ringing
Action: Increase spatial resolution, reduce interface contrast
Trade-off: Increased scan time and prolonged breath-hold

Central point artefact

This artefact appears as a focal dot of increased signal within the centre of an image. Typically the scanner vendor will have installed software to prevent this and a call to the service representative is required if this artefact is noted.

Summary

Aetiology: Failure of DC correction software
Appearance: Focal dot of increased signal in centre of image
Action: Call scanner service representative

Conclusion

CMR can:

    1. Provide invaluable anatomical and functional cardiovascular assessment in a safe, noninvasive manner free from ionizing radiation, and using contrast agents with low nephrotoxicity;

    2. Be used in patients with prosthetic heart valves, sternal wires, joint replacements, retained epicardial pacing leads, and intracoronary stents.

CMR cannot:

    Replace echocardiography.

Further reading

Short breaks

Physics

Schild HH. *MRI made easy (...well almost)*. Germany: Heenemann, 1990. Sponsored by Schering AG.

Clinical

Pennell DJ, Sechtem UP, Higgins CB, Manning WJ, Pohost GM, Rademakers FE, et al. Clinical indications for cardiovascular magnetic resonance (CMR): Consensus Panel report. *Eur Heart J* 2004;25:1940–65.

Combination

Mohiaddin RH. *Introduction to cardiovascular magnetic resonance*. UK: Current Medical Literature, 2002. Sponsored by Servier. This book is highly recommended for the clinician.

Longer haul

Physics

Mitchell DG. *MRI principles*. USA: WB Saunders, 1999.

Combination

Manning WJ, Pennell DJ (eds). *Cardiovascular magnetic resonance*. USA: Churchill Livingstone, 2002.

Index